School Health
Programs

Other books by Dean F. Miller

A Bibliography of Environmental Health Literature Available in the Toledo, Ohio, Area

SCHOOL HEALTH
PROGRAMS
Their Basis in Law

DEAN F. MILLER

South Brunswick and New York: A. S. Barnes and Company
London: Thomas Yoseloff Ltd

A. S. Barnes and Co., Inc.
Cranbury, New Jersey 08512

Thomas Yoseloff Ltd
108 New Bond Street
London W1Y OQX, England

Library of Congress Cataloging in Publication Data

Miller, Dean F
  School health programs.

  Bibliography: p.
  1. School hygiene—Law and legislation—United States.
I. Title.
KF3826.S3M5   344'.73'0794   79-39349
ISBN 0-498-01158-5

Printed in the United States of America

This book is dedicated to my wife,
Karen, who as a wife and a
mother has never been found "liable"
or "negligent" and to our two
children, Barbara Jo and Brian.

Contents

List of Tables

Preface

The author's interest in school administration and school law has led to the writing of this book. Since many decisions that a school administrator is called upon to make involve matters relating to some phase of the school health program, it becomes apparent that there be proper understanding of legal principles affecting the school health program for the purpose of providing direction in the decision-making process. Identification and application of the legal bases which guide the practices existing in the school health program are of importance to all school personnel. All personnel, whether directly involved in the school health program or not, need to have some understanding of the legal bases of their programs. Those activities of the school health program which are governed by legislative statute, administrative rules and regulation, court decisions, or attorney general's opinion must be apparent to any school personnel involved in a decision-making situation.

The importance of the foregoing concepts first became apparent to the author during his early teaching years and was reemphasized upon his thinking during graduate study. Often the question was raised as to "what is the law?" with regard to some problem or question under consideration. Seldom was there found a single source that could be used in resolving such problems and questions. Realizing this from personal experience and having had opportunity to become involved with school administrators and teachers of all grade levels through workshops and in-service projects, the value of knowing the legal bases governing decision-making in matters relating to the school health program has led to the writing of this book.

It is hoped that those who find themselves in a decision-making situation relative to some problem relating to the school health program will find this volume helpful. It must be understood that numerous administrative rules and regulations unique to a particular state or local school district must be known and applied by any school administrator. These rules and regulations are far too numerous to include in this volume. It is highly possible that all of the legal principles discussed will not be applicable to school personnel in every state. However, this book should serve as a general reference to any person regardless of the locality of his school.

Encouragement for writing this volume has been given by numerous individuals with whom the author has had opportunity to speak regarding the subject matter contained herein. Also, the author's wife has rendered extensive encouragement and help by proofreading each section and offering positive and helpful grammatical corrections. For this I am deeply appreciative.

D.F.M.

1
School Health and
School Law

In the American educational system numerous programs
have been developed through the years. The school health
program is a very important aspect of any educational
program. It is this program that seeks to provide experiences
for school children that will positively effect their physical,
emotional, and social well-being.

The school health program consists of three broad areas.
These areas or phases are known as: 1) *the health instructional program,* sometimes referred to as the school health
education program, 2) *the school health services,* and 3)
the provisions for a healthful school environment.

The instructional phase of the school health program
includes the identification of specific behavioral objectives
and subsequent provision of learning experiences for the
child in relationship to the identified objective. These learning experiences may be in either the cognitive, effective,
or affective domain.

The school health services are those activities performed
by the school or under the direction of the school for the

15

purpose of contributing to the health and well-being of each child. Activities for appraising the child's health are included. Such appraisal may be accomplished by vision and hearing screening, periodic medical examinations, and direct teacher observations for deviations from the normal. Provisions for controlling communicable disease and for providing emergency services for the sick or injured child are a part of the health services rendered by the schools.

Since a child spends a rather significant portion of each school day in the school environment, numerous factors contribute to his health and well-being. Such factors as proper lighting, proper acoustics, proper sanitation, a good water supply, and heating and ventilation are all important to the health of the school child. Because children must be transported to school in many areas of the country, the school bus transportation program is also important. The provisions for eating lunch, and in many places breakfast, also contribute to the child's school performance.

Many practices of the school health program have their bases in law. These legal bases may be found in statutory provisions. Each state has some statutory provisions which give direction to the school administrator regarding particular aspects of the school health program. Another source of legal basis rests in the administrative rules and regulations of the state or local board of education. A third source of legal direction comes from those legal principles established by court decision as a result of litigation. All personnel involved in the school health program and in school administration need to have some understanding of the legal bases of this very important program.

A body of legal matters which affects the various phases of education has developed. This is known as *school law.* School law includes all the rules and regulations that pertain to education. School law is the application of general legal principles to the conduct of school activities.

School law, as is true of all law, is in a constant state of change. It is very clear that a school administrator must be knowledgeable with respect to school law and its changing status. There are numerous statutes and principles of law that affect many of the school administrator's decisions and actions, regardless of one's administrative or supervisory responsibilities. Many of the decisions that a school administrator makes have legal foundation of which he may be unaware. Not only in the school health program, but in all aspects of the educational program, the school administrator must understand and apply those laws and regulations which pertain to his school and to those people under his responsibility, both employees and students. *Every school administrator, as well as teacher, should be acquainted with the broad area of information known as school law.*

All rules and regulations which relate to education are a part of school law. School laws should serve as tools to the school administrator in directing the total school program. These laws should give direction to the school administrator by informing him of what he must do, what he may do, and what he cannot do.

The legislative branch of government produces the statutes and laws for a specific state. *Statutory laws* come from the legislative processes. Some statutes are found to be mandatory, while others are of a permissive nature. Many statutory provisions only specify minimal standards which often the school administration is willing to accept as maximal.

Legislative statutes are not perfect. A particular statute may be misunderstood with regard to the specific intent and operation of the law. These misunderstandings lead to differences of opinion, interpretation, and conflict in applying legislative statutes to specific cases. Such conflicts and misunderstandings must be resolved by the courts. The branch of government which has resolved these conflicts and misunderstandings by process of law is the judicial branch. From court decisions come the establishment of precedents and guidelines which are known as *common law*.

The judicial courts do not merely interpret the laws. In addition to interpreting laws where the legislature has presented a statute, the courts will, when no law exists, make a ruling and establish a precedent for future similar cases.

The courts have established various rulings on the principle of *stare decisis*. The principle of *stare decisis* has been defined as:

> Doctrine that, when court has once laid down a principle of law as applicable to a certain state of facts, it will adhere to that principle, and apply it to all future cases, where facts are substantially the same. . . . When point of law has been settled by decision, it forms precedent which is not afterwards to be departed from.[1]

It is not possible to develop statutes for every situation. For this reason, the decisions of courts have become important. It has been the responsibility of the courts to interpret existing statutes and to determine solutions to problems arising out of litigation for which there was no statute or for which the statutes might have been confusing or contradictory. If no statute exists which applies

1. Henry Campbell Black, *Black's Law Dictionary* (St. Paul, Minn.: West Pub. Co., 1951), pp. 1577–78.

to the facts as presented before a court, the court is then forced to look to other courts for guidance. The decision reached is based upon the precedents established by previous court cases. These previous interpretations are usually adhered to by other courts of law.

School law has helped to establish a framework for rules and policies within the school. Because of the increase in school litigation in recent years, an understanding of school law has become increasingly important to both school administrators and to the teachers. To be ignorant of one's legal obligations as a leader in education could result in many problems. Ignorance of the legal obligations might result in extended court actions. These court actions could lead to extensive financial expenses, as well as an unnecessary expenditure of time and energy. Also, negative publicity, bringing discredit to the persons involved, could result from a lawsuit. Unawareness of legal obligations may cause a school administrator to become personally involved in a lawsuit.

Many litigations in our courts of law which concern the schools or school employees have involved the health and well-being of the students. Byrd has stated, "the administrator has a professional obligation to know the basic elements of school health law and to see that legal requirements and responsibilities are enforced."[2] Many legal requirements and principles of law have been established from court decisions which relate to the school health program.

When the question is raised, "What is the law?" with regard to a certain practice in the school program, it is important that one know what the *source* of the law is in addition to what the law says.

---

2. Oliver E. Byrd, *School Health Administration* (Philadelphia: W. B. Saunders Co., 1964), p. 43.

Summary

The school health program is an integral part of any school curriculum. This program consists of three phases: health instruction, health services, and provisions for a healthful school environment. Many activities of the school health program have their bases in law. These legal bases are made up of various rules, regulations, statutes, and legal opinions. This body of knowledge is known as school law. School administrators must be aware of those legal principles which relate to the various phases of the school health program.

2
Legal Research Methodology

Most school personnel, administrators, supervisors, and teachers have had no experience with legal reference material or methods. Seldom in the research training of the school person is reference made to methodology in legal research. Yet to be an effective administrator in understanding school law, some familiarity with the material, methods, and procedures of legal research is necessary. An acquaintance with the literature and materials available for doing legal research is very useful. The school administrator needs some familiarity with the law library so that he can go directly to the sources of law and seek answers to questions which may arise. Legal resource material is of a primary and secondary nature.

Primary Sources

Primary sources of law are the state statutes and decisions rendered by courts of law. Notz has stated that "in any legal research, statutory law should be located first and then court decision."[1] Drury and Ray, when referring to the research worker in school law, emphasized the same point by stating that an individual "in embarking on his research to find the answer to a question of school law, first consult the statutory law of the state with which he is particularly concerned."[2]

Statutory law is best located by going directly to the records of the acts themselves or to an annotated edition of the statutes. In addition to an annotated presentation of the statutes, these records usually contain a history of the law, including amendments to the law and notations about any repealing action that has occurred. Citations to court cases in which the particular law has been mentioned are given. Also, any opinions of a state attorney general which have been rendered for the purpose of clarifying some point of law relating to the specific statute are included in an annotated listing of the statutes.

The attorney general of a state is the legal advisor to the executive officials of the state government. An attorney general's written opinions are advisory statements and not mandatory orders. Even though the opinions and rulings of an attorney general are not mandatory or legally binding, they are very persuasive. They normally are followed by governmental officials and by the courts in ruling on court cases. In most cases, an attorney general's opinion will clarify particular questions of law raised with respect to some point of law. The attorney general of the state may wish to render an opinion for the purpose of clarifying a statute or court decision. These opinions help in legal

1. Rebecca Laurens Love Notz, *Legal Bibliography and Legal Research* (Washington, D.C.: National Law Book Co., 1947), p. 91.
2. Robert L. Drury and Kenneth C. Ray, *Principles of School Law* (New York: Appleton-Century-Crofts, 1965), p. 326.

research work by giving further understanding as to what the intent of the given law is and what its meaning is in actual practice. The opinion is usually expressed in answer to a specific question.

Decisions that have been rendered by the courts are very important primary sources in the establishment of various principles of law. It is important to consider court decisions at all levels of government. Federal, state, and local court decisions all play a role in establishing principles of law.

There are two kinds of index books for locating court cases. These references are digests and encyclopedias. A legal digest presents an index which is classified by subject. Encyclopedias present by topic a narrative statement of the law with footnote references to specific cases.

Probably the most extensive series of legal digests is *The American Digest System.* This digest system covers every federal, state, or local case reported in the United States since 1658. There are 419 topics arranged in alphabetical order within this digest. Other digests that are valuable in locating court cases are regional digests, such as the *Northwestern Reporter Digest,* and state digests. One other source of court cases in digest form is the *American Law Reports* series.

Several legal encyclopedias give a comprehensive listing of court decisions on different topics. *Corpus Juris* and *Corpus Juris Secundum* are legal encyclopedias which contain listings of court decisions on over four hundred different topics. Statutory law is not covered in these legal encyclopedias. Court cases or citations of authorities with reference to a particular principle of law are included.

Another important legal encyclopedia is *American Jurisprudence.* Volume 47 of *American Jurisprudence,* Volumes

78 and 79 of *Corpus Juris Secundum,* and Volume 56 of *Corpus Juris* deal specifically with legal topics of concern to the schools and school districts.

Once a person has found a court case appropriate to the subject of concern, he can read the record of the case in the *National Reporter System.* The *National Reporter System* includes all the cases from courts of record in the United States and contains the opinion or opinions of the court in rendering its decision. Cases decided by the United States Supreme Court, as well as federal cases which come before the Federal Circuit Courts of Appeals, are included in the *National Reporter System.*

The *National Reporter System* includes opinions of state appellate and trial courts and of the federal courts. There are seven regional reporters and four federal units.

In reading a court case, the facts surrounding the situation should first be determined. From this understanding of the facts, the issues with which the court had to deal are established. Then the decision of the court is presented including reasons suggested for the particular ruling which has been given. The facts, issues, decision, and pertinent reasons presented for the decision should be identified. Cross-reference should then be made to all similar cases to determine what reasons were given by the court in each situation in reaching its decision in answer to the issues raised. After determining the reasons presented by the court for its decision, the principle of law basic to the situation is ascertained.

In order to determine if later cases followed, modified, disapproved, or reversed the decision handed down by the court of record, *Shepard's Citations* should be used. From *Shepard's Citations* it is possible to determine if any changes have resulted since the original decision was rendered. In addition, one can see what other legal decisions have been based on the case at hand.

Secondary Sources

Numerous textbooks and reference books are available which serve as secondary sources of information relating to school law. One of the most inclusive is the *Yearbook of School Law* edited by Dr. Lee O. Garber. This publication is printed annually and contains a résumé of court decisions which deal with court litigations involving the schools. Publications by such organizations as the National Organization on Legal Problems in Education and the National Education Association relating to school law are valuable secondary sources of legal information for the school administrator.

Definitions

Legal research work demands not only a grasp of the procedures, literature, and materials, but also familiarity with the language, terms, and phrases unique to the legal profession. The following are words or phrases often found in legal material that must be understood by any person doing research work in school law.

Court decision: The judgment handed down by the court after all arguments are heard. This decision is the ruling of the majority of judges hearing the case.

Court of record: A court which has a permanent record kept of its acts and proceedings.

Defendant: The person against whom a suit is being brought.

Et al.: An abbreviation for *et alii,* meaning "and others."

Et ux.: A legal abbreviation meaning "and wife."

Ex rel.: Legal proceedings on behalf of another.

Legal opinion: The statement by a judge or court of the decision reached in regard to a case tried or argued, expounding the law as applied to the case and detailing the reasons upon which the judgment is based.[3] Either a concurring opinion or a dissenting opinion may be presented. A concurring opinion agrees with the decision, but wishes to emphasize some point; a dissenting opinion is an expression of reason for not agreeing with the final decision.

Litigation: A contest in court.

Plaintiff: The person who claims to be injured. It is this person who brings suit against another to obtain a remedy for supposed injury to his person or property.

Statute: A law enacted by an appropriate legislative branch of government.

Supra: Refers to a previous reference.

Summary

School personnel often have little familiarity with legal reference literature and procedures of legal research. Legal resource material is of a primary and secondary nature. Primary sources of legal material include records of statutory acts, attorney generals' opinions, digests, encyclopedias, and the actual records of litigation found in the *National Reporter System.* Once a court case has been found and read, it is necessary to properly brief the case. From the study of the facts, issues, decision rendered, and reasons

---

3. Henry Campbell Black, *Black's Law Dictionary* (St. Paul, Minn.: West Pub. Co., 1951), pp. 1243–44.

presented by the court for its decision, principles of law basic to the particular situation can be identified.

Secondary sources of legal material are widespread and can render extensive help to the school personnel seeking guidance in solving many school problems. This source material includes books, journals, periodicals, monographs, and numerous other publications.

3
School Health Instruction

The phase of the school health program which includes direct teaching and learning experiences and activities affecting one's health behavior is known as health instruction. This phase of the school health program includes separate class periods for presentation and study of various health concepts. Health often is included in the school curriculum as is any other academic discipline. Health instruction many times is correlated into other subject matter areas such as general science, physical education, home economics, and the social sciences. In the elementary grades, health concepts may be integrated in activities and units as they fit into the various problems being studied.

School districts are free to include in the school curriculum any subject not prohibited by state constitution or state statute. Every state in the United States except two (Alaska and Delaware) has at least one statute pertaining to some aspect of health instruction. Statutory requirements relating to health topics rank second only to those pertaining to the teaching of history and government. Historically, when some factor or factors have arisen which created a specific health problem, there has been a tendency to pass a law requiring the schools to take action to counteract the problem. This has been seen as recently as the concern over drug abuse and related legislative attempts to deal with this problem. In our nation the educational curriculum is responsive to the will of the public. What the people seem to feel is important often has found its way into the school curriculum.

Massachusetts was the first state to legally require any teaching of health or health-related subjects. In 1850, the teaching of physiology and hygiene in all of the public schools of Massachusetts became a legal requirement. Much of the support for and interest in such a law was a result of the interest in health related matters in the school curriculum by Horace Mann, the first secretary of the state board of education in Massachusetts.

In the years following, many other states passed statutes requiring that physiology and hygiene be taught in the schools. Late in the nineteenth and the early part of the twentieth century, partially as a result of the efforts of the Women's Christian Temperance Union and other pro-prohibition organizations, many states passed laws requiring some instruction about alcohol, tobacco, and narcotics. Many of these laws are still on the statutory books today.

There are numerous state statutes relating to instruction in health areas. These statutes vary considerably from state to state. Some health education related topics found in state statutory provisions are: 1) physiology and hygiene, 2) alcohol, tobacco, and narcotics, 3) health and physical education, 4) nutrition, 5) dental hygiene, 6) sanitation, 7) fire prevention, 8) safety, 9) sex education, and 10) critical health problems.

Of all the statutory requirements relating to health education, instruction concerning alcohol and narcotics is required in the greatest number of states. Table 1 presents a list of those states in which state statute requires teaching about alcohol and narcotics. Forty-four of the fifty states require such instruction. In Illinois no teacher can be certified, according to state statute, who has not passed an examination relating to alcohol and narcotics. According to this law, not only is the teacher to pass an examination covering content knowledge relating to alcohol and narcotics, but the teacher is to be able to make a presentation of the best methods of teaching this material. The state of Maine has a requirement that no elementary teacher will be certified unless evidence of training in physiology and hygiene with special reference to the effects of alcohol, stimulants, and narcotics can be presented. Minnesota law says nothing about requirements prior to certification. However, all students in teacher preparation curricula must have course work in the effects of alcohol and narcotics on the human system, on character, and on society. Similar requirements concerning certification and satisfactory performance on examinations with reference to alcohol and narcotics are found in New Jersey and New York. The New Jersey law exempts music, art, and manual training teachers from this requirement.

TABLE 1 *States Requiring Teaching about Alcohol and Narcotics*

Alabama	Nevada
Arizona	New Hampshire
Arkansas	New Jersey
California	New York
Colorado	North Carolina
Connecticut	North Dakota
Florida	Ohio
Georgia	Oklahoma
Idaho	Oregon
Illinois	Pennsylvania

Indiana	Rhode Island
Iowa	South Carolina
Kentucky	South Dakota
Louisiana	Tennessee
Maine	Texas
Massachusetts	Utah
Michigan	Vermont
Minnesota	Virginia
Mississippi	Washington
Missouri	West Virginia
Montana	Wisconsin
Nebraska	Wyoming

Health, as an academic subject, is required in sixteen states. Table 2 presents a listing of those states with requirements for the inclusion of health in the school curriculum. Often this requirement is to be given in combination with physical education, according to the statute.

TABLE 2 *States Requiring Instruction in Health Education*

California	Maryland	Ohio
Georgia	Maine	Oklahoma
Idaho	Minnesota	Rhode Island
Iowa	Montana	Vermont
Kansas	Nebraska	
Louisiana	New Jersey	

Physiology and/or hygiene is required in twenty-one states. Usually this requirement has an additional statement attached to the wording of the law emphasizing the inclusion of instruction relating to alcohol and narcotics. Most of these requirements have their derivation many years ago.

TABLE 3 *States Requiring Instruction in Physiology and/or Hygiene*

Alabama	Mississippi	Pennsylvania

Colorado	Missouri	Rhode Island
Illinois	Montana	South Carolina
Iowa	Nevada	Utah
Maine	New Hampshire	Virginia
Massachusetts	New Jersey	Washington
Minnesota	North Dakota	Wisconsin

Statutory requirement for instruction in safety education is found in sixteen states. Table 4 presents a listing of the states with such a requirement.

TABLE 4 *States Requiring Instruction in Safety*

Arkansas	Mississippi	Pennsylvania
California	New Jersey	South Carolina
Connecticut	New York	Tennessee
Illinois	Ohio	Virginia
Maryland	Oklahoma	Wisconsin
		Wyoming

Ten states mandate some instruction relating to fire prevention. These states are: Arkansas, California, Nebraska, New Jersey, New York, Ohio, Rhode Island, South Carolina, West Virginia, and Wisconsin.

In examining the legal bases for the health instructional phase of the school health program, the role that various court decisions have played in influencing the school curriculum must be considered as well as the statutory requirements. In relation to the other phases of the school health program, there has been little litigation directly concerning health instruction. The authority of the school board to require pupils to study specific subjects in the school curriculum has seldom been tested in the courts. It generally has been assumed that the state has the right to make whatever curricular requirements it so desires regarding subjects in the school curriculum. Since attendance at school is compulsory in all of the states, it has been the opinion of the courts that the state could require certain courses as part of the school curriculum. No court case or reference to a court case can be found in which the court ruled against the inclusion of a specific subject in the school curriculum as long as the course was approved by either the state and/or the local board of education.

A principle of law supported in an Indiana case[1] upheld the concept that a school board may require a pupil to take a particular subject in the school curriculum, regardless of whether the parents object. In this case, the school board adopted a regulation requiring all high school pupils to study music. The father of one student objected and the student was expelled from school. The court refused to issue a *writ of mandamus* requiring that the student be reinstated. The court supported the school board regulation requiring that a specific subject, in this case, music, be a part of the school curriculum for all students. Therefore, it can be assumed that requiring the instruction of any particular subject, such as health, is a proper and legal responsibility of a school board.

Not only may a school board require that a certain subject be included in the school curriculum, but it would appear that the courts may decide what content should or should not be included in the particular course of instruction. This has occurred very infrequently, but such legal precedent has been set. In a case in New York,[2] an elementary school student was injured doing a headstand in a physical education class. The courts ruled that this was an unreasonable exercise for a student at this grade

1. State *ex rel.* Andrews *v.* Webber, 108 Ind. 31, 8 N.E. 708 (1886).
2. Gardner *v.* State of New York, 256 App. Div. 385, 10 N.Y.S. 274 (1939).

level. In rendering this decision, the court was decreeing what content could or could not be taught in the physical education curriculum. It could be a dangerous precedent to permit the courts to determine content within the educational curriculum as a result of legal opinions rendered by the courts.

Occasionally, questions have arisen concerning the excuse of students from various aspects of the health instructional program because of religious beliefs. State statutes requiring specific instruction in certain areas of health education usually are accompanied by a provision giving permission for excuse from such instruction by presenting written request to the proper school authorities. A second legal principle bearing on this subject has been established by the courts in rulings which deal with immunization and vaccination cases. In these cases, the courts have consistently ruled that certain statutes making vaccination and immunization a requirement before a child may enroll in school are constitutional and not against the basic principles of religious freedom as set forth in the United States Constitution. For this reason, many cases probably are not brought to court because the weight of evidence as to how the courts would decide the cases already is available in the decisions rendered regarding vaccination and immunization.

A ruling with respect to a question involving participation in physical education class established a principle that in all likelihood would carry the weight of law in a court case involving objection to health instruction. In a case in 1962,[3] the court ruled that a student, on religious principles, was not required to participate in certain objectionable exercises in the physical education class. Neither

---

3. Mitchell v. McCall, et al., 143 So. 2d 629 (Ala., 1962).

was this pupil required to wear the standard physical education uniform. However, the pupil was obligated to attend the class, excluding the mentioned objectionable activities. The implication for health instruction would seem to indicate that if objection were raised to certain parts of the instructional program, such as sex education or other controversial topics, a child could be excused from that part of the program which was objectionable. However, blanket excuse would not seem to be possible unless permitted by statute.

Sex Education

Curriculum workers have attempted for some time to incorporate in the curriculum of the school experiences relating to human sexuality. This has taken the form of various approaches and involved several academic disciplines. Various names have been given to such educational experiences: "sex education," "family life education," and others. The 1960's saw development of numerous sex education programs throughout the United States.

Extreme opposition to programs of sex education arose in 1968 and 1969. Many varying procedures were used by those in opposition in an attempt to force school boards to remove from the curriculum learning experiences relating to human sexuality and reproduction. State legislatures reacted by passing statutes relating to this matter. The courts were called upon to render decisions challenging the legality of such programs.

The Michigan legislature identified what it perceived sex education as being:

Sex education is the preparation for personal relationships

between the sexes by providing appropriate educational opportunities desgined to help the individual develop understanding, acceptance, respect, and trust for himself and others. Sex education includes the knowledge of physical, emotional and social growth and maturation, and understanding of the individual needs. It involves an examination of man's and woman's roles in society, how they relate and react to supplement each other, the responsibilities of each towards the other throughout life and the development of responsible use of human sexuality as a positive and creative force.[4]

Upon legally defining sex education, the legislature authorized school districts the permissive right to hire instructors to teach sex education. School districts had the authority to provide facilities and equipment as needed for this instruction. The statute made it clear that instruction relating to socially deviant sexual behavior was to be a part of the curriculum.

The Michigan Department of Education has the responsibility to aid in establishing programs of sex education. The department is to establish a library of films, tapes, and other literature to be used in this program. Such supplies are to be made available to schools as they develop their courses. The statute also stipulated that the Department of Education is to aid the colleges and universities of Michigan in establishing in-service programs for teachers who will be teaching in the sex education curriculum.

Provision for exemption from the program is given when parents or guardians present a written notification of their desire that their child not participate. No penalty is to be given, either by grade reduction or graduation requirements, to those who request to be excused.

In 1965 the Illinois legislature passed a Sex Education Act. This Act established a Division of Sex Education in

4. Michigan, P. A. 1968, No. 44

the office of the Superintendent of Public Instruction. A Sex Education Advisory Board was also established.

Authorization was given in this act to establish programs of sex education throughout the state. As in the Michigan statute, the Illinois provision gave authorization for the establishment of programs in state universities for training teachers in this very delicate subject matter area.

In 1969, as the result of opposition to sex education programs in Illinois, another statute was passed suggesting that no pupil would be required to take sex education if their parents submit written objections. If the parents wish to examine the instructional materials being used, they must be given the opportunity to do so.

The Louisiana legislature passed a law prohibiting any one from teaching sex education in an elementary or secondary school of that state. Not only is instruction forbidden but no text, quiz, or survey is to be conducted regarding personal beliefs or practices in sex, religion, or morality. The provisions of this statute also apply to non-public schools.

The law is to be in effect until a legislative study committee appointed in 1969 presents its report. This committee was to make recommendations designed to strengthen educational support of the family structure and good moral character. Advice was to be sought from various sources.

A Tennessee statute passed in 1969 makes it unlawful to teach sex education unless such courses are approved by the state and local board of education. Any courses in sex education are to be taught by qualified teachers. The determination of qualification is left to the local school board. This statute does not apply to high school courses in biology, physiology, health, physical education, or home economics.

The state of California legislature passed a law making it unlawful to require students to attend classes in which human reproductive organs and their functions and processes are described, illustrated, or discussed. If such a class is held, the parents are to be notified in writing. The parent may request in writing that his child not attend the class. Such a request for exemption is valid for one school year, even though the child may personally want to participate.

All parents are to be notified that they may preview any written or audio-visual material to be used in the course. The statute does not apply to descriptions and illustrations of human reproductive organs in physiology, biology, zoology, general science, or health science textbooks.

In litigations involving sex education courses, the courts have ruled in favor of the programs. Citing one case in Maryland,[5] suit was brought seeking to prevent the sex education program. The suit challenged a board of education decision to provide a comprehensive family life and sex education program in every elementary and secondary school. This program was to be a part of the health education program.

The litigants claimed the board's ruling violated their right under the First Amendment and two clauses of the Fourteenth Amendment (Equal Protection Clause and Due Process Clause). They held that parents have the exclusive constitutional right to teach their children about sex. This right was to be performed in the home, and they contended it prohibited teaching sex in the schools. Their opposition to the sex education program based on the First

5. Cornwell v. State Board of Education, 314 F. Supp. 340, affirmed 428 F. 2d 471 (Md., 1969).

Amendment was supported by the concept that such instruction would lead to the establishment of religious concepts.

It was pointed out that the state board of education has responsibility to determine the educational policies of the state and to enact laws necessary for the administration of a public school system. Such school board regulations have the force of law. Therefore, this ruling relating to sex education was found to be neither unreasonable nor arbitrary.

The court found the position of the plaintiffs to be without merit. No legal authority could be found to support the contention that parents have exclusive right to teach their children about sex. It also was the opinion of the court that the purpose of this school board ruling was not to establish any particular religious dogma. The court considered the ruling as a public health measure, pointing out that the legal principle has developed which suggests that as part of the police power of the state, interest in the health and welfare of citizens outweighs claims based upon religious freedom.

Therefore, the motions of the plaintiff were dismissed and the court stated the following:

> There would appear to be . . . reason for the State Board to provide sex education for the non-pregnant (and, incidentally, for the non-impregnating) as for those students who, because of a lack of information on the subject (or for other reasons), have become pregnant or who have caused pregnancy.[6]

In Hawaii, in 1968, the state legislature approved an education department proposal to provide instruction in

6. *Ibid.*, 314 F. Supp. 342.

the area of social problems. Family life and sex education was to be included in this program. A curriculum was adopted for the fifth and sixth grade. Included in the curriculum planning was a film series entitled, "Time of Your Life."

Suit was brought challenging the program,[7] claiming it was an invasion of one's privacy and a violation of one's religious freedom. The plaintiffs felt that only parents should have the right to teach sex intimacies to their children. A related complaint was that such instruction infringed upon the parents' rights to educate their children in sexual matters pursuant to their particular religious beliefs. Particular objection was raised to parts of the "Time of Your Life" series dealing with: 1) The Male, 2) The Female, 3) A New Life, 4) Questions Please, and 5) Growing Up.

Children were not required to attend the classes. No compulsion or coercion was placed upon students to be involved in the program. Also, the parents were provided an opportunity to preview the materials that were to be used.

The court ruled in favor of the sex education program, pointing out its belief that one's right of privacy had not been violated in this case. Also it was felt that the sex education program in no way infringed upon the parents' right of practice of religious freedom.

The importance of permitting children to be excused from such programs, if the parents object, cannot be over-emphasized. In New Jersey,[8] the state board of education has a regulation requiring attendance at a course entitled

---

7. Medeiros v. Kiyosaki, 478 P. 2d 314 (Hawaii, 1970).
8. Valent v. New Jersey State Board of Education, 274 A. 2d 832 (N.J., 1971).

"Human Sexuality." According to the regulation, no one is to be excused on grounds of personal conscience from this course.

The regulation was challenged by parents claiming that it violated the First, Ninth, Tenth, and Fourteenth amendments. The position of the local school board regarding this matter was that if a child could be excused from this course, then one could object on grounds of conscience to many other required activities in the school program.

The objection of the parents was upheld and the policy was ruled to be unconstitutional. It is important to note that the inclusion of the course in the school curriculum was not ruled unconstitutional, but the policy of not permitting students to be excluded on religious or other grounds was considered to be illegal.

It can be seen that there is sound legal basis for establishment of sex education programs as long as the statutory requirements of the state are adhered to. Provision should be made for exclusion of students whose parents object, and it would appear to be legally sound to permit parents to preview material that will be used in the course. Possibly such a practice, though time consuming, should be referred to as "adult education." Maybe the parents will find their own ignorance being replaced by sound sex education concepts.

Drug Education

In recent years, the increase of drug abuse has led many agencies to examine their role in helping to combat this problem. Much attention has been directed to what the schools can do. Research has been conducted, commissions and committees formed, projects developed, and many other procedures taken in order to come to some plan for counteracting the growing drug abuse problem.

At the legislative level, several states have passed legislation directing the schools to become more specifically involved in this area. For years all but a few of the states have had statutory requirements making teaching about alcohol and narcotics and their effects on the human body a necessity. However, since medically most drugs of abuse are not narcotics (such as the hallucinogens, barbiturates, and amphetamines), it is doubtful how effective these older statutes are in giving direction for today's drug abuse problems.

The most specific state legislative requirement is the one passed in the state of Montana. Specific dates for implementation were written into this provision. By July 1, 1972, every state university in Montana and all private colleges which have course work in teacher preparation must establish a course for credit in health education which will include instruction in drug abuse and alcohol education. By this same date, all secondary schools must teach a course in health education with the same emphasis on drugs and alcohol. This same provision made it mandatory that for any teacher in the state to be certified after December 31, 1972, he must have successfully completed the health education course stipulated in the law.

In Florida a Drug Abuse Education Act was passed in 1970. Barbiturates, hallucinogens, narcotics, alcohol, and tobacco were included as drugs of concern in this act. The act called for a comprehensive K-12 program of drug education in the schools of Florida. Several priorities were established. In order to have well qualified teachers, in-service education for upgrading teacher knowledge was identified as one priority. Another called for the development of various resource centers for aiding the schools by providing films, educational materials, and other instructional media for teaching the drug courses. The act encourages the development of drug education courses in the state institutions of higher education.

Provision was made for exempting any student from this instruction whose parents objected because of religious beliefs. A very interesting paragraph in this act said that nothing in this statute should be construed to authorize or to require the teaching of *sex education*.

The Michigan state legislature passed a Critical Health Problems Education Act in 1969. Drugs, narcotics, and alcohol were identified as critical health problems to be dealt with. In addition, several other content areas were listed. They included tobacco, mental health, dental health, vision care, nutrition, disease prevention and control, and accident prevention.

This act provides for in-service programs for training teachers. Emphasis was placed on encouraging better preparation in health education at the college level in the content areas identified. The act also provided for the development of health curricula relating to the critical health problems.

Miscellaneous

Several states have statutory provisions which are unique to that particular state. Because of the interest in ecology and man's environment in the past couple of years, at least two states (Florida and California) have passed legislation making it mandatory to incorporate instruction in this area in the school curriculum.

In 1970 the California legislature amended a statute requiring the instruction of school children in personal and public safety and accident prevention, fire prevention, and health by including the provision for teaching about the protection of our environment in the school program.

The Florida legislature, in the same year, passed a provision creating an environmental education program. This statute is to encourage coordination of various disciplines concerned with the environment. Special concern was expressed in the law for urban environmental problems.

One of the most unusual statutory provisions is found in Wisconsin. Realizing that Wisconsin is known as the "dairy state," it is quite easy to see the vested interest resulting in this requirement. Instruction is to be provided in all schools, both public and private, in the true and comparative vitamin content of dairy products. The food and health values of dairy products are to be studied with emphasis being given to their importance in the human diet. The statute says such instruction is to be given in elementary schools as well as in high school.

Various states have requirements for setting aside specific days or weeks for emphasis on topics that relate to health. One week during the school year in South Carolina is to be designated Alcohol Education Week. From the sixth grade through high school for at least thirty minutes on each of three days, instruction is to be given concerning the risks and dangers involved in the use of alcoholic beverages. One assembly of not less than forty-five minutes is to be devoted to alcohol education during this week.

Several states have a requirement that Temperance Day be observed in the schools. Various provisions and recommendations are specified, all with emphasis on studying about temperance. The specific day set aside varies. In

Maine it is to be the first Friday in March. In Georgia, the fourth Friday in March shall be devoted to teaching at least for two hours in all schools the good of temperance and the evils of intemperance. January 16 is to be Temperance Day in the state of Washington. North Dakota and North Carolina also have days set aside as Temperance Days. As would be expected, all of these statutes were written into law in the latter part of the 1910's and the early part of the 1920's.

One other day set aside by legislative provisions can be found in Nebraska. The first Friday in November is to be known as State Fire Day. At this time various exercises and instruction are to take place appropriate to this subject.

Missouri and North Dakota have statutory laws requiring that instruction be included about tuberculosis. Hawaii has a mandatory provision that dental hygiene instruction be included in the school curriculum.

Summary

The legal bases for much of the health education (instructional) program are to be found in statutory regulations. Since the first statutory requirements in Massachusetts in 1850, there have been numerous and varying laws developed relating to different aspects of the health education program throughout the United States.

Principles of law established by court decisions have not been as common, nor as extensive, with respect to this phase of the school health program as in the other two phases. Common law has established the principle that school boards may require the inclusion of whatever subjects in the school curriculum that they desire, as long as state constitution or state statute does not prohibit. This makes it possible for the inclusion of health instruction in the school curriculum.

The content to be included in the health instructional program varies from state to state. These differences in content are determined by statutory requirement, as well as by administrative rules and regulations. State and local boards of education present innumerable requirements relating to health instruction. The magnitude of administrative rules and regulations relating to health instruction is too extensive for complete inclusion in this presentation.

Common law has made provision for exclusion of children from certain aspects of the school instructional program which are found to be in conflict with one's religious beliefs. This question has been raised recently with regard to teaching sex education. Yet sex education has been ruled to be constitutional and legal, the same as any other content area of the school curriculum.

4

School Health Services

Most states have some statutory requirements relating to the school health services. A majority of these provisions mandate what the schools are to require concerning immunization and vaccination of the school child. Many provide guidance to the school administrator in controlling communicable and infectious diseases.

More court litigations have resulted in the various school health services than either of the other two phases of the school health program. Not only must statutory requirements and administrative regulations be known in analyzing the legal bases of the school health services, but, also, the principles of law established and rendered through court decisions and legal opinions should be understood.

The concept of the role of the school health services in the school program has broadened in recent years. At the turn of this century the school health services consisted mostly of emphasis on sanitation of the school and on control of communicable diseases through vaccination, immunization, and isolation. Today, the school health services are much more inclusive and exhaustive.

The courts have recognized the importance of the school

47

health services and have ruled consistently in favor of the school in litigations brought against various aspects of this school program. As early as 1910, a court in Minnesota recognized the importance of the school health services by stating:

> Education of a child means much more than merely communicating to it the contents of textbooks. . . . The physical and mental powers of the individual are so interdependent that no system of education, although designed solely to develop mentality, would be complete which ignored bodily health. And this is peculiarly true of children whose immaturity renders their mental efforts largely dependent upon physical conditions. It seems that the school authorities and teachers coming directly in contact with the children should have an accurate knowledge of each child's physical condition, for the benefit of the individual child, for the protection of the other children with reference to communicable diseases and conditions, and to permit an intelligent grading of the pupils.[1]

Consideration of the emergency care procedures and the requirements for immunizations and vaccinations will be discussed in later chapters.

School Health Service Personnel

In order for a school district to have an effective health service program, personnel must be employed to fulfill various responsibilities. The classroom teacher cannot be held responsible for every part of the health services as they relate to the school child. School nurses, physicians, dental hygienists, and dentists are the personnel most commonly employed by school boards to provide health

---

1. State *ex rel.* Stoltenberg *v.* Brown, 128 N.W. 295 (Minn., 1910).

services in a school setting. One state, Virginia, authorizes through statutory provision the using of school funds for employment of physical therapists. In addition to authorizing employment of a physician, nurse, dentist, and dental hygienist, New York has a law permitting employment of an oculist and a nutritionist by local school boards.

There have been attempts to prohibit the schools from employing physicians, nurses, and dentists. The courts have ruled that unless restricted from doing so by statute, a school board may hire these people for work in the health service program of the school.

An extended opinion was presented by a court in Kentucky[2] expressing the rationale as to why a nurse was considered an appropriate individual to be hired by the school board. In this situation, the school board created a new position and hired an individual to fill the vacancy. The created position was a combination school nurse and teacher of health and physical education. The creation of this position by the school board was challenged in court. After hearing the case, the court ruled that hiring of a nurse and teacher of health and physical education was legal. In the supporting opinion, the following discussion was presented:

It is not alone the duty of the home to build in the child the purpose of self-direction in respect to its physical welfare. It is the duty of the school which the child attends, every year, during the greater portion of its youth, which is not of its own choosing, under conditions and circumstances not of its own making, to build in the habits and life of such child self-direction in respect to its physical well-being. Its health and physical development while in school are essential and

2. Board of Education of Bowling Green v. Simmons, 53 S.W. 2d 940 (Ky., 1932).

indispensable, not only to the child's mental development, but to the conduct and success of the school. Its actual health and physical condition should be of no less concern to the governing authority of the schools than its mental growth.

Several services that the school nurse may render effectively for the betterment of the school child were suggested by this court. These services were: 1) detection and prevention of communicable diseases, 2) immunization of pupils, 3) discovery of physical defects among school children, 4) emphasis on community and personal hygiene, 5) aid in and promotion of the physical development of all school children, and 6) supervision of the school health program.

The court further pointed out that the school nurse was considered to be in a category different from that of other teachers. As such, regulations controlling certification of teachers were not applicable to the school nurse. The nurse should not be required to meet the same standards for certification as the teachers because she was not expected to render the same kinds of services as was a classroom teacher.

This concept has caused other court litigations to result. The status of the role of the school nurse has been questioned several times in court. The New Mexico Supreme Court[3] concluded that a nurse does not have the same status as a teacher or as any other school employee who is certified to teach. However, this court did not state an opinion as to its concept of the role of the nurse or the status of such an individual within the school program.

More recently this same legal principle has been upheld

3. Bourne v. Board of Education of City of Roswell, 46 N.M. 310, 128 P. 2d 733 (1942).

in California.[4] In establishing a school employee salary schedule, a different maximum salary was set than that which was applied for teachers. The salary schedule for the school nurses was the same as the teachers until a certain level was reached. At this level the nurses' salary became "frozen," whereas the teacher would continue to receive annual salary increments.

Two nurses already had salaries in excess of the newly proposed maximum level. The board was ordered by a lower court to apply the salary schedule for all certified personnel to the two school nurses. The school board appealed the lower court decision, claiming that the nurses were in a distinct class of certified employees, apart from the teaching staff.

The Court of Appeals reversed the original judgment. This decision was based on the concept that the salary schedule as adopted was not an arbitrary act. It was ruled to be permissible and legal. The decision was based on the legal principle that a school board has the power to classify certified employees differently according to training, experience, and duties.

It is important that medical personnel employed by the schools be used for screening, appraisal, and examination purposes only. Court decisions have suggested that medical personnel must not render medical or surgical treatment as part of their school-related responsibilities. The Supreme Court in Colorado was very emphatic in noting that school personnel were not authorized to render medical or surgical treatment to the school children. The court ruled that the school district could employ personnel to conduct health inspection programs but nothing more. The court stated:

---

4. Eastham v. Santa Clara Elementary School District, 76 Cal. Rptr. 198 (1969).

The board may provide for the physical as well as the mental education of the pupils. It follows that, if they provide physical education, they must, within reasonable limits as to expense and time of pupils, provide for determining what is proper and beneficial for each pupil, by all reasonable means, including examination, physical as well as mental, . . . This should not include medical or surgical treatment for disease. That would be to make infirmaries or hospitals of the schools.[5]

Medical Examinations

Medical examinations have been a very important part of the school health services for many years. These examinations have been conducted by school physicians, as well as by the students' family physicians, for the purpose of appraising the health status of the child. The medical examination is thought of as an educational experience for the child, as well as a screening device. Medical examinations are given as fulfillment of requirements for admission to school, to detect various communicable diseases, for athletic participation purposes, and for various other reasons. It is very common to require all students newly enrolled in a school district to have a medical examination prior to beginning classes.

The regulation that each student must have a medical examination prior to being admitted into any school within a particular school district for the first time falls under the principle of the police power of the state. In requiring such an examination, the schools are helping to protect the health and welfare of the public by making sure no diseased child enters school.

In many states there exists some statutory authorization

5. Hallett, *et al. v.* Post Printing and Publishing Co., 192 P. 659 (Colo., 1920).

for requiring medical examinations of school children. These laws usually indicate who must submit to the medical examination and when this requirement must be fulfilled. Provision usually is established in the statute for excluding those students who object, or whose parents object, because of religious beliefs.

In the absence of contrary legislation, the school board has the authority to require a medical examination of children as a prerequisite for admittance to school. This principle was challenged in 1914 in South Dakota.[6] Suit was brought against a local board of education having a regulation which required that each year all pupils in the school, before being admitted, must have a medical examination. This examination could be conducted by the family physician at the expense of the parent, or it could be conducted by the school physician at the expense of the school district. The results of this examination were to be filled out on a physical record card furnished by the school.

Two children, whose parents objected to the physical examination because of religious beliefs, did not provide the health cards and were not admitted to the school. Suit was brought against the school board by the parents of the children. In the suit, the parents contended that the school board had no authority to require a physical examination before admitting the children to school on the grounds that no authority was conferred on the local board by the state statute for such a regulation. The regulation was challenged, arguing that the medical examination might cause such mental suggestion of disease, so as to cause an actual disease.

The court ruled that the school board did have the

6. Streich *v*. Board of Education of Independent School District of City of Aberdeen, *et al.*, 34 S.D. 169, 147 N.W. 779 (1914).

right to enforce such a regulation. The court ruling was based on the principle that police power is necessary for self-preservation. The police power of the state permits the state to prohibit all things harmful to the comfort, health, and welfare of society. The regulation was not invalid on any points raised by the parents. The requirement was a reasonable regulation to ask of all school children.

From this case, a definite principle of law concerning requirements of medical examinations for students has been established. This principle affirms the authority of a school district, in the absence of a state statute, to require a medical examination as a prerequisite for admittance to school. This principle is applicable in the absence of legislation to the contrary.

In Texas,[7] a school district hired nurses and doctors for the purpose of examining and then instructing the students concerning their health condition. Physical examinations were conducted for all students. Women physicians examined the female students, and male physicians examined the boys. If the parents or guardians of the children objected to the examination by writing to the school principal, their children were not examined. Parents and guardians were encouraged to be present at the examination. A written record with recommendations was kept for each child. The school nurses and doctors were not to treat any of the children except in situations requiring emergency care. The parents were encouraged to employ their own physicians for the purpose of treating defects found during the examination at school.

Suit was brought against the schools, claiming that by conducting a medical examination of all children at school,

7. Moseley, et al. v. City of Dallas, et al., 17 S.W. 2d 36 (Tex., 1929).

a health department was being operated. This department, it was alleged, was operated and conducted by the school board in the public schools, and the expenses for its operation were being paid out of school funds. The court supported the conducting of medical examinations as a legal part of the total school program. It was the opinion of the court that the operation of this program did not constitute the operation of a health department. In upholding the program of giving medical examinations to children at school, the court stated:

> Modern science has conclusively established the fact, and the record in this case conclusively shows, that there is an intimate relation between the mind and the body, and no teacher can intelligently deal with the child's mind who ignores such child's physical condition. It therefore follows, as a matter of course, that money wisely and judiciously expended by the school board within proper limitation to ascertain the child's physical condition is a wise and legitimate expense of the teaching process.[8]

Not only may medical examinations be required of the students, but they also may be required of school teachers and administrative personnel. In New York,[9] an assistant principal was informed that she must have a physical examination. She refused and was reassigned to another job in the school system. Her new job was an administrative assistant in the curriculum department. Her salary was the same in the new position as in the former. However, in the new position she did not come into contact with students as was the case in the position of assistant principal. In court this former assistant principal sought to restrain

8. *Ibid.,* p. 41.
9. Kropf *v.* Board of Education of City of New York, 238 N.Y.S. 2d 757 (1963).

the school board from enforcing the regulation that she must have a physical examination. The court upheld the school board ruling that teachers and school personnel could be required to have periodical medical examinations.

If a teacher should fail to pass a physical or psychological test, what should the school board do or what is it required to do? The only possibility is to release the individual. Such actions have been contested in court. In New York,[10] school board rules and regulations, even to the point of being able to release teachers on grounds of physical or emotional disabilities, are legal. It is very important if a school board is forced to take such action that sufficient evidence is available to show that the teacher is incompetent due to the physical or psychological reason.

This same principle was supported in another case in New York City.[11] A teacher had applied for a regular teaching license but was rejected. This individual had a record of a heart condition in his medical history. For six years the teacher had served as a regular substitute teacher. At the time of his initial licensing, a one year certificate, he declared that he had an aortic stenosis (narrowing of the artery). An aortic valve did not function as it normally should because of calcification.

Three years after the initial licensing an artificial valve was placed in the heart to replace the damaged aortic valve. Three years after the operation this individual's personal physician stated that the aortic function was now normal and that other heart difficulties were no longer of concern. Supporting evidence was also rendered from the hospital.

---

10. Corlov v. Nyquest, 304 N.Y.S. 2d 486 (1969).
11. Corsover v. Board of Examiners of City of New York, 298 N.Y.S. 2d 757 (1968).

However, the examining physician for the school district would not approve the application because of "heart disease." Normally when a conflict arises between the report of a physician employed by a school district and the private physician, the courts have ruled in favor of the school district. However, in this case, the school district physician presented no objective medical findings to support the decision to refuse a teaching certificate. The court ruled that the school medical authority's findings must be overruled and the proper teaching license should be issued.

As seen in statutory requirement, the most common concern of school personnel in requiring medical examinations is the detection of persons with active, positive reactions for tuberculosis. About one-half of the states have some statutory provision requiring periodically either a chest X ray or a skin test for tuberculosis. In some states this is an annual requirement; in others it is required every two or three years.

Occasionally, the question has arisen as to whether the school district may stipulate in its regulation that the medical examination must be conducted by a medical doctor. Unless provided for by statute, it would appear that the schools must accept reports from chiropractors and osteopaths, as well as medical doctors. This was noted in a 1965 case in Colorado.[12] In this situation, the Colorado Supreme Court ruled that the schools must accept an examination report by a chiropractor. The school district had refused to accept a chiropractor's certificate of examination. The parents of the child filed suit, claiming that the chiropractor's report met the regulation requiring a medical examination to be given before the child could be enrolled

12. Flemming v. Colorado State Board of Education, 400 P. 2d 932 (Colo., 1965).

in school. In ruling upon this case, the court supported the position of the parents. The opinion of the court was stated as follows:

> Chiropractors are licensed and regulated by the State . . . Through similar statutes medical doctors and osteopathic physicians are accredited. Chiropractic is defined . . . as among the healing arts, . . . the authorized practice includes diagnosing, analyzing and treating human ailments. Chiropractors are subject to examination in the basic sciences in the same manner and to the same extent as are all others—medical doctors and osteopaths—in the healing arts.[13]

Medical examinations are an important aspect of the school health services program. It must be remembered that no provisions should be made for the treatment of illnesses and physical defects found as a result of the medical examinations by school personnel unless authorized by state statute.

In West Virginia, state statute authorizes school districts to maintain dental clinics. These clinics are to be used for the teaching of oral hygiene and for providing treatment of defective teeth if such is requested by the parent or deemed necessary by the board of education.

State statute in Pennsylvania requires a dental examination to be conducted by a school dentist three times in the child's school experience. This dental examination is to be given once upon the child's original entrance to school and again in the third and seventh grades. The school is to provide space for these examinations and the parents of the children are to be notified of the results. Provision is made in this law for accepting a report from the family dentist in lieu of the school examination.

---

13. *Ibid.,* p. 935.

Oregon law authorizes a dental care program. Any school district with at least a student population of one hundred thousand may conduct a dental health program. Such a program is to provide facilities for dental examinations or treatment. Those who cannot pay are to be given free care. No one is to be required to receive the dental examination.

School Health Records

Most schools keep some kind of health records for each pupil. Occasionally, the question has arisen as to whether these school health records can be made available for inspection.

In determining if the school health records can be examined, state statutes, as well as published administrative regulations and rulings of the local school district, must be known. The right of parents and other interested persons to inspect the health records of school children must be examined in light of statutory directions and administrative regulations and rulings. If no statute or administrative regulation is available, common law must serve as the guide.

It is generally assumed, unless otherwise prohibited by statutory requirement or administrative regulation, that the right of inspection of public records, including the school records and school health records, is permissible. However, very little judicial precedent has been established concerning this point. This right is subject to certain limitations. The main limitation in such a situation rests in the determination of whether the individuals wishing to examine the records have a special interest in and reason for seeing the specific health records.

The determination of whether the health records of a university student could be examined was not answered directly by a court in Texas.[14] This court was of the opinion that health records can be examined if they fall within the legal definition of *public records*. If the health records are public records, an individual has the right to inspect his own health records. The question of what is a public record is a matter for which each court must rule.

No direct ruling has been given indicating whether the school health records can be considered as legal public records. However, a court has ruled that scholarship records of pupils in public schools are to be considered legally as public records[15] and as such, are available for the inspection of certain interested persons.

In 1961, in New York,[16] the courts ruled on a case concerning the right of a parent to inspect the school records of his child. In this case, the school recommended that a boy was in need of psychological treatment and therapy. The father had the family physician write to the school for an abstract of the records of this boy. The school psychologist forwarded the needed records. The father also requested a copy of his son's records. The request of the father was refused by the schools. The boy's father then brought court action against the school, requesting that all of his son's school records be made available to him.

Testimony in this case pointed out that there was no statute available either giving permission to or prohibiting a parent from inspecting the school records of his child. Under further investigation, the court ruled that there was no legal reason why the parent could not inspect the

14. Morris *v.* Smiley, *et al.*, 378 S.W. 2d 149 (Tex., 1964).
15. Valentine *v.* Independent School Dist. of Casey, *et al.*, 174 N.W. 334 (Iowa, 1919).
16. VanAllen *v.* McCleary, 211 N.Y.S. 2d 501 (1961).

health records of his son. The court stated that "a parent is entitled to inspect the records of his child maintained by the school authorities." Since no constitutional, legislative, or administrative permissions or prohibitions could be located, the father's petition to examine the records was granted.

Much the same ruling was established in another case in New York City.[17] The court ruled that the parents could examine the records under the condition that such examination and inspection must take place at the school board office. The parental examination and inspection of the school health records must be observed and supervised by an authorized school official.

Another accepted legal principle quite widely held by the courts is that the right to inspect records commonly carries with it the right to copy the information on the record. Prudence must be used in permitting individuals to examine the school health records of school children. However, school health records should be released only to those persons who have a definite interest in the child and a reason to see the records. These records should be made available only on a "need to know" basis.

Exclusion from School and Readmission to School

The question has often arisen as to when a child must be excluded from school because his presence is detrimental to the well-being of other students. In many states determination of this procedure is set forth in the state statutes. Most state statutes relating to this problem require that a child with a contagious disease be sent (or taken) home

17. Johnson v. Board of Education of the City of New York, 220 N.Y.S. 2d 362 (1961).

and not permitted to return until he is free of the infectious microorganisms. Some states do not have statutes which provide for all possible situations, and many statutes are somewhat nebulous regarding this point. Therefore, situations have arisen from time to time when the courts have been called upon to resolve such questions.

If there is any question as to the possibility that a child may be carrying an infectious organism, the courts have supported the schools' actions in excluding the child from school. In North Dakota, in order to prevent the spread of trachoma, a local board of health required that the school board deny admission to the public schools of all children affected with or suspected of having trachoma.

Suit was brought in this situation in which parents sought permission for their two children to attend school. One of the children had been refused admittance because a physician and federal health service officer found the child to have trachoma. The other child was refused admittance because it was suspected that he had trachoma; however, no signs or symptoms were present. The question was raised in court as to whether the children really had trachoma or some other disease. Regardless of what they had, the North Dakota Supreme Court ruled that such exclusion was reasonable. The court concluded its opinion by stating:

> The seriousness of the disease and its communicable character afford ample foundation for such an order; . . . this discretion should not be exercised in a way that might result in needlessly exposing healthful children to a disease as serious as trachoma.[18]

Another legal principle established from court decision is that children may be excluded from attendance at school after having some communicable disease until a medical

18. Martin *v.* Craig, *et al.*, 173 N.W. 788 (N.D., 1919).

certificate is presented, giving proof that the child is no longer infectious. In Minnesota, a student was sent home from school with a sore throat and a throat infection. There was a strong possibility that this student had diphtheria. The school district required that before the girl could be permitted to return to school, it would be necessary for her to present a certificate from a physician verifying that she no longer had an infection. The student's parents objected to this requirement on religious grounds. They claimed that the girl was well and that no epidemic was present at this particular time. For this reason, it was their contention that there was no need for requiring a certificate from a physician.

This ruling of the school board was challenged by the parents in court. The Supreme Court of Minnesota upheld the school board regulation. In presenting the legal opinion upon which the court decision was reached, the court stated:

> We must recognize that one child may quickly spread a disease among the many children it comes in contact with in school. It seems more reasonable to us to have the rules applicable in preventing as well as controlling an epidemic. . . . These rules do not really exclude any one except by his own volition. The record in this case merely placed before plaintiff a condition to his child's admission to the school. The condition required is a certificate of a physician, and, in case of sore throat or suspected diphtheria, a negative report from a culture submitted to the division of public health.[19]

This decision supported the legal principle that children can be excluded from school until a medical certificate is presented, giving proof that the child is no longer infectious. The court made the point in stating its opinion that the teacher in no way was qualified to tell if the infection was

---

19. Stone *v.* Probst, *et al.*, 206 N.W. 644 (Minn., 1925).

still present. Only a physician could make this determination.

A case in Arizona[20] involved a situation where all students were prohibited from attending school. The local board of health passed a resolution declaring that all schools must be closed because of a Spanish influenza epidemic. The school board questioned whether the board of health could do this. The school board claimed that there were no epidemic conditions present at the particular time. It was their contention that over eighty per cent of the students were free of the disease and could attend school. For this reason, the school board maintained that the board of health regulation was not needed. However, the court ruled that the regulation was reasonable as a proper measure for protecting the health of the public. This board of health ruling was to be in force only during the time of the epidemic. The principle of law upon which this court based its decision was that when the board of health felt conditions were such that the schools should be closed for the health and welfare of the public, it had the right to order such action unless prohibited from doing so by statute.

Today there seems to be a different philosophy in public health work concerning closing of schools during the time of an epidemic. Complete closing of schools usually is not accomplished when epidemic conditions are present. However, the principle established in the Arizona case, that the local board of health had the legal *right* to prohibit persons infected with a highly communicable disease from attending school until the individual no longer was a potential source of infection, still carries the weight of law in many areas of the country.

---

20. Globe School District No. 1, of Globe, Gila County *v.* Board of Health of City of Globe, 20 Ariz. 208, 179 P. 55 (1919).

Any statutes, regulations, or administrative rulings calling for specific procedures in excluding or readmitting students from school are established for the health, safety, and welfare of the public. Such regulations normally will be upheld by the courts. School board rulings and regulations must always be examined in light of the statutory provisions applying to the specific situation.

Summary

Legal direction relative to the school health services is very extensive. Most states have statutory provisions regarding various aspects of this phase of the school health program. Litigation has been quite extensive and numerous legal principles have been established. Even though some of the litigation is rather dated, the principles of law are important to the school administrator.

The courts have upheld the practice of a school district's employing medical personnel. Their responsibilities are: 1) to appraise the health status of the students, 2) to render emergency care, and 3) through consultation to guide the students to the place where the needed medical attention can be received.

If a child is felt to have a communicable disease or some other contagious condition, the schools may exclude the child from attendance. Readmittance policies should be determined by the school district. The burden of responsibility for such determination of readmittance should not rest with the classroom teacher, but with a medical physician.

The school should keep records relating to the health of a school child. Such records should be made available to those who have reason to use the information.

5
Torts, Negligence, and Emergency Situations

School districts often have no written policies available outlining what is to be done if an injury or illness should occur to a child during the school day. Many times school personnel will refrain from providing the needed care because of fear of possible resulting litigation. There is great variance in practice as to how emergency conditions are handled by school personnel. Before one can discuss the legal implications of rendering emergency care to a sick or injured child in school, several important concepts must be understood.

Torts

If, as the result of one's actions, an injury occurs to another individual, a tort has been committed. Not only might the injury or damage be done directly to the person, but it might be an act directed against his property. A tort can be committed either through an act of omission

66

or an act of commission. Common torts may be acts of negligence, acts of trespass, assault and battery, defamation of character, or the maintenance of a nuisance.

Negligence

Negligence has been defined many times by the courts and in legal reference material. Black has described negligence as "the omission to do something which a reasonable man . . . would do, or the doing of something which a reasonable and prudent man would not do."[1] Negligence has been the most common type of tort liability. The most frequent basis for bringing suit in matters pertaining to negligence has centered around cases where personal injuries have resulted. Matters involving negligence have very important implications for the school health environment phase of the school health program and for the school health services.

Under the legal system in the United States all people have a right to expect freedom from bodily injury caused by another person. Negligence can only be an issue when an injury has occurred. It must be proven that some act of negligence has taken place which resulted in an injury.

School employees are responsible for the health and welfare of the students who come to school. The relationship between students and school personnel is one of *in loco parentis*. This means that the school employee is serving in the place of the parents.

One of the earliest court decisions with respect to the principle of *in loco parentis* stated in 1837:

---

1. Henry Campbell Black, *Black's Law Dictionary* (St. Paul, Minn.: West Pub. Co., 1951), p. 1184.

When parents in fulfilling their duty of training their children into useful and virtuous members of society, place them in charge of a school-teacher for the purpose of acquiring certain forms of education, by that fact the school-teacher becomes in Loco Parentis in regard to all matters pertaining to that particular phase of the child's life which is entrusted to his guidance for development, including the power and duty of correction.[2]

This relationship has placed much more responsibility on the school teacher or administrator than what would ordinarily be expected of a normal individual. For this reason, Burt suggested that it would be more accurate to define negligence, as it pertains to the school teacher, as "the failure to act as a reasonably prudent *teacher* would act in the same or similar circumstances."[3] A greater degree of care and responsibility should be expected from a teacher than from a person not in the teaching profession.

Foreseeability

Foreseeability has been particularly important in matters involving school personnel. The first and often main test to determine if negligence was involved has been a test of foreseeability. The test has been used to determine if one's conduct were reasonable and proper or if the individual were acting in a negligent manner. The test lies in determining whether the person has taken those "foreseeable" precautions that would be expected of a normal person to prevent potential accident situations from occurring. One must anticipate and prevent those situations

---

2. State *v*. Pendergrass, 19 N.C. 349 (1837).
3. Lorin A. Burt, *School Law and the Indiana Teacher* (Bloomington, Ind.: Beanblossom Publishers, 1967), p. 62.

from developing which might be dangerous to the students. It is vitally important that the school principal and teacher constantly be looking for potentially dangerous conditions involving the school program.

Defenses against Negligence

An individual charged with committing a negligent act has several defenses which he may employ. Any one or a combination of several may be used as a defense against charges of negligence.

In a court of law, the plaintiff must show that the negligent act was the direct and immediate cause of the injury. This is known as the defense of *proximate cause* or as it is sometimes referred to, the legal cause. Proof must be exhibited that negligence was the direct and actual cause of injury. The plaintiff must have an actual loss or damage to himself or to his property as the result of the action with which he is confronting the defendant.

The plaintiff not only must prove negligence, but he must show the court proof that the injury would not have happened except for the proven act of negligence. The Supreme Court in Nebraska has upheld this legal defense and has stated:

> It is a fundamental rule of negligence that to be actionable the negligence charged must be the proximate cause of the injury. In other words, the negligence must be such that the accident would not have occurred but for the existence of the negligence charged.[4]

A second defense against negligence is a *vis major* or

4. Odom *v.* Willms, 131 N.W. 2d 140 (Neb., 1964).

an act of God. If an injury has occurred as the result of an event which is beyond the control of human beings, then the defendant is not negligent. Such occurrences as a storm, lightning, tornado, and earthquakes are examples of natural happenings which would serve as legal defenses against negligence. The influence of man can do little to protect against harm and injury under these circumstances.

3rd A third defense against negligence is *assumption of risk*. Any activity entered upon in life entails some risk. Assumption of risk is the voluntary participation into an activity which is potentially dangerous. This defense against negligence has been particularly important with regard to injuries obtained in physical education and athletic activities.

An individual participating in sports and games or any other normal school activity assumes some degree of risk. However, the courts have not always permitted this defense to stand as a defense against negligence. Even though a person might voluntarily enter into a potentially dangerous activity, he may not fully understand or adequately be instructed in the dangerous aspects of that activity. The activity may be inherently dangerous, yet the instructor is considered to be negligent if he has not made for equality of competition by size and ability or if he has not informed the students of the dangers involved and instructed them in the proper safety precautions.

4th A fourth defense against negligence is *contributory negligence*. Each individual has a certain responsibility for his own safety and protection. Any conduct of a person which falls below that standard he would normally be expected to maintain for his own self protection is contributory negligence.

The legal defense of contributory negligence is very important to the school principal or school teacher in the elementary grades. The basis for determining contributory negligence has been to determine if the actions of the plaintiff were actions that would be expected of a normal person of similar age, maturity, and ability. The younger the individual, the less responsible he can be held, legally, for his own self-protection. It is extremely important that greater precautions be taken when working with younger children or inexperienced adults.

Governmental Immunity – *Public Agency cannot be held negligent for tort liability.*

A common law principle that has special implication for the schools and school personnel is the common law doctrine of governmental immunity. The doctrine of governmental immunity states that a public agency cannot be held negligent for tort liability. Only if it consents to being sued, can an agency of the state be brought to court. The concept that the sovereign received his power by divine right led to the idea that the "king could do no wrong." For this reason, an agent of the government could not be held for his torts and be brought to trial unless out of benevolence he consented to do so.

The doctrine of common law immunity originated from English case law. It generally has been assumed that the doctrine of governmental immunity had its origin in the case of Russell *v.* The Men of Devon.[5] In this case, Russell sued the male inhabitants of the County of Devon for damages to his wagon as the result of a bridge being out of repair. It was the responsibility of the county to maintain such structures as the bridge. However, the court ruled against Russell. The court stated the beliefs, with

5. Russell *v.* The Men Dwelling in the County of Devon, 100 Eng. Rep. 359, 2 Term Rep. 667 (1788).

respect to the abolishment of the common law rule of immunity, that:

1. To permit it would lead to "an infinity of actions."
2. There was no precedent for attempting such a suit.
3. Only the legislature should impose liability of this kind.
4. Even if defendants are to be considered a corporation or quasi-corporation there is no fund out of which to satisfy the claim.
5. Neither law nor reason supports the action.
6. There is a strong presumption that what has never been done cannot be done.
7. Although there is a legal principle which permits a remedy for every injury resulting from the neglect of another, a more applicable principle is "that it is better that an individual should sustain an injury than that the public should suffer an inconvenience."[6]

The origin of the common law doctrine of governmental immunity in this country was established in Massachusetts in 1812.[7] A horse was drawing a stagecoach on a road between New York and Boston. In the town of Leicester the road passed over a stone bridge in need of repair. There was a large hole between the stones on the bridge. When crossing the bridge, one of the horses pulling the stage-coach stepped into the hole. The horse fell and the stagecoach passed over his body. The horse later died, and the owner sued the city claiming that the inhabitants of the community were negligent in the maintenance of the bridge.

The court, upon hearing the case, held that by common law ruling the public agency could not be held liable. It

6. Lee O. Garber and E. Edmund Reutter, co-editors, *The Yearbook of School Law: 1964* (Danville, Ill.: The Interstate Printers and Publishers, Inc., 1933-1971), pp. 235–6.
7. Mower *v.* The Inhabitants of Leicester, 9 Mass. 247 (1812).

was ruled that the government of Leicester was a quasi-corporation created by legislature for purposes of public policy and as such was considered to be subject to common law. Unless provided for by statute, the state could not be held negligent based upon the common law ruling established in the Russell *v*. Men of Devon case. Since this ruling was presented, the common law doctrine of governmental immunity has been the law of the land in the courts of the United States except where overruled by statute or struck down by court decision.

The common law doctrine of governmental immunity has been criticized as being unjust. For years there has been criticism of and objection to the application of this doctrine as it pertains to public officials. As early as 1929, the *Indiana Law Journal*, commenting editorially on the case of Forrester *v*. Somerlott, reported:

> That the school corporation is an agent of the State seems unquestionable; that the State is not liable for negligence of its officers and agents is undoubtedly the rule of Indiana; but that the doctrine of State irresponsibility should be the law is, on principle, very questionable. This doctrine, based on a theory of State sovereignty, has its roots in the now exploded belief in the divine right and prerogative of kings. . . . The modern trend of legal philosophy seems to be toward treating the State as a personality and holding it liable for its torts the same as an individual.[8]

Many legal scholars have been of the opinion that the doctrine of governmental immunity is no longer appropriate in our society. In recent years the trend has been toward a more liberal view in our courts. This liberal viewpoint

---

8. "Schools and School Districts—Negligence—State Liability for Torts," *Indiana Law Journal* (February 1929). 4:343.

has given less prestige to the doctrine of common law immunity than it had been given previously.

The traditional belief of those who accept the common law doctrine of governmental immunity has been that it was a misapplication of public money to make payment for individual injuries. The liberal viewpoint has suggested that the cost of injuries should not be borne by only one person or a few people, but should be shared by many in the society. According to the United States Constitution, compensation must be made for taking or damaging of private property. The liberal thinker has reasoned that it is inconsistent that a governmental agency cannot damage or take private property without some compensation; yet under the doctrine of governmental immunity, an individual can injure or destroy another's person or property without liability being ruled and without the possibility of the injured individual receiving compensation.

Another reason often given for justification of the doctrine of governmental immunity is that the school district receives no advantage from operating the schools; therefore, they should not be charged with liability. The idea has often been held that the personal interest of an individual must give way to the concept of the public good.

The courts have been reluctant to deviate from this common law doctrine of governmental immunity unless told to do so by the legislative body through legislation. In the view of most courts, it is the responsibility of the legislature, not the courts, to change the rules. This was expressed in 1943 by an Oregon court, when it was stated:

It may be that the common-law rule of immunity is harsh and unjust in requiring the individual alone to suffer the wrong in the instant case, and that society, in keeping with the modern trend, should afford relief, but this is a legislative and not a judicial question.[9]

In 1959, the Illinois State Supreme Court overruled the common law doctrine of governmental immunity in the case of Molitor and the Kaneland School District.[10] In this case involving an injury to a child as a result of an accident on a school bus, the Illinois Supreme Court stated that the whole purpose of the Revolutionary War and of the Declaration of Independence was to abolish the divine right of the kings in the United States. Hence, the opinion was rendered that the common law doctrine of governmental immunity was no longer applicable in Illinois. This was the first time that a court in the United States ruled against the law of governmental immunity.

Since then, several states have ruled against the common law doctrines of governmental immunity. In those states where the concept of governmental immunity still is in force, quite often the school district has been found to be immune, but the individual employee of the school board can be held liable for acts of negligence. Since much variation exists from one state to another and even some discrepancy exists within a state, a school administrator must know the current status of the doctrine of governmental immunity within his particular state.

Liability

As the result of the doctrine of governmental immunity,

9. Lovell v. School District No. 13, Coos County, 143 P. 2d 236 (Ore., 1943).
10. Molitor v. Kaneland Community Unit District No. 302, 163 N.E. 2d 89 (Ill., 1959).

the school, in serving as a governmental agency, has been considered to be immune from tort liability.

A point of consideration as to whether a school district is immune from suit lies in determining what functions were being performed at the time of the injury. Often the courts have ruled that the schools are free from liability if they are involved in a governmental function. A governmental function includes activities commonly associated with the responsibility of the government. Such functions as police and fire services, welfare services, and education have been considered governmental functions. School functions usually have been classified as governmental functions by the courts.

However, if the function is a proprietary function, the school district may be found liable. A proprietary function is an activity not governmental in nature. The function can be performed by a company or by a private citizen. If an activity is conducted for the sake of profit, the rule of immunity is not in effect, as an activity which is profit-oriented is considered a proprietary function.

The Supreme Court of Pennsylvania in a 1964 ruling[11] on a case where charges of negligence were brought against an employee of a school district said, "This Court has always applied the rule that a School District is not liable in trespass for the negligence of its officers and employees while engaged in *governmental* functions." The implication of this statement is that school districts will be held liable if the injuries are the result of negligence in a proprietary function.

The determination of whether a function is governmental or proprietary in nature is exceedingly difficult. According to most courts, a school district seldom performs a proprie-

11. Supler *v.* School District, 182 A. 2d 535 (Pa., 1962).

tary function. The courts have ruled that the purpose of schools is for the education of the students. This is a governmental function and, according to the Tennessee Supreme Court, there is no such thing as a school district acting in a proprietary capacity.[12]

In further support of this viewpoint, the courts have ruled that sports events at which admission is charged are governmental functions.[13] Likewise, the operation of a school cafeteria has been declared a governmental function.[14]

Emergency Care

Any individual rendering emergency care to a sick or injured person will find that suit can be brought against him for acts that may have been committed in the process of helping that individual. The converse of this is also true. Failure to provide some help when necessary may result in a case of negligence. This situation rests on the tort principle of omission, a person not acting to help the sick or injured individual. No matter what action an individual takes, he is liable for his actions, whether they be acts of omission or acts of commission.

Even though it is true that a person may be found negligent for performing an act of emergency care or for not rendering assistance, most feeling concerning giving of emergency care to a sick or injured person seems to be that any care which is reasonable and which is performed with no hope of personal gain usually will not result in an adverse decision being rendered against the individual.

12. Reed v. Rhea County, 225 S.W. 2d 49 (Tenn., 1949).
13. *Ibid.*
14. Elias v. Norton, 4 N.E. 2d 146 (Ohio, 1936).

A principle of law which has been applied to various cases is that one is expected to render such care as a normally prudent person would exercise under similar circumstances. The Supreme Court of Indiana expressed this concept as follows:

> Where one is confronted with a sudden emergency, without sufficient time to determine with certainty the best course to pursue, he is not held to the same accuracy of judgment as would be required of him if he had time for deliberation. Accordingly, if he exercises such care as an ordinarily prudent man would exercise when confronted by a like emergency, he is not liable for an injury which resulted from his conduct, even though another course of conduct would have been more judicious, or safer, or might even have avoided the injury.[15]

Legal questions have arisen regarding rendering emergency care to school pupils. It seems that the teacher has a legal responsibility for rendering aid to any student who becomes injured or sick while under the supervisory care of the particular teacher. This concept has arisen out of the principle of law which states that teachers are acting *in loco parentis* in relation to the students. The rationale of this concept implies that parents would be expected to care for their children if they became injured or were sick. Failure to do so would be considered negligent action on the part of the parent. Since the teachers, during the time the students are at school, are serving in the place of the parents *(in loco parentis)*, they must be considered to have a legal responsibility to aid any sick or injured student.

This concept raises a number of questions that must be resolved by school administrators. Since training in emer-

15. Gamble, *et al. v.* Lewis, 85 N.E. 2d 634 (Ind., 1949).

gency care procedures (first aid) is seldom a prerequisite for employment by a school district, the legal status of the school administration in hiring a teacher not qualified to perform emergency care comes into question. No litigation is presently available which would give direction on such a matter. It would be hoped that school administrators would take proper steps to avoid the possibility of litigation involving emergency procedures.

Since it is a legal responsibility of the teacher to come to the aid of a sick or injured student, the question of what kind of aid and how much is expected of the teacher must be examined. Usually, the circumstances and the ability of the teacher dictate what should be done. A legal principle which has been upheld often by the courts with respect to administering emergency care to a sick or injured person by a teacher or school employee has been:

> The standard of care required of an officer or employee of a public school is that which a person of ordinary prudence, charged with his duties, would exercise under the same circumstances.[16]

The particular circumstances surrounding the situation usually are weighed very heavily in cases involving injury to students at school. The importance of determining what is ordinary care depends upon the circumstances of the particular case. A court decision rendered in a litigation in California said that ordinary care is to be determined with reference to "the situation and knowledge of the parties."[17] The basis for rendering a decision lies with a

16. Lehmuth v. Long Beach Unified School District, et al., 343 P. 2d 428 (Calif., 1959).
17. Lilienthal v. The San Leandro Unified School District of Alameda County, 293 P. 2d 891 (Calif., 1956).

jury. Such a decision is to be given based upon evidence as to whether the teacher rendered reasonable care.

In situations where injury does occur under the supervision of school personnel, it is important that prompt emergency care be obtained. This concept can be seen by examining a decision rendered as the result of litigation in California.[18] A boy was injured in a game of touch football during the noon hour. The injured boy had blocked a boy larger than himself. The knee of the larger boy struck the injured player's abdomen. His spleen and one kidney were injured and eventually required removal by surgery.

The injured boy was taken immediately to the first aid room and covered with a blanket. About two hours later, the instructor asked the boy to pass urine. Blood was observed in the urine. The instructor than took the injured boy home.

The father later sued the school district on the grounds of improper supervision of the activity and for failure to give prompt attention to the boy. The court did not render a decision favorable to the injured boy in this case. As the case developed, the question of lack of supervision was quickly and easily disproven. However, the question concerning prompt medical attention was considered. It was the testimony of a medical expert that a layman cannot be expected to discover internal injuries except by observing certain external signs. In this situation, the external sign of the internal injuries was the passing of blood in the urine. Therefore, until this sign appeared, the layman could not have been expected to know there were injuries to the spleen and the kidneys. Medical authority felt that

18. Pirkle *v.* Oakdale Union Grammar School District, City of Oakland, County of Stanislaus, 253 P. 2d 1 (Calif., 1953).

no injury resulted during the time the boy was resting in the first aid room.

The implication developed, from the opinion rendered, that there is a responsibility on the part of school personnel to provide prompt emergency care when pupils are injured. That care which is to be rendered is to be within the framework of the knowledge, the training, and the understanding of the signs and symptoms of the conditions of the injured individual.

In New York,[19] a boy was accidentally kicked in the head during his physical education class and died of resulting skull fracture. Suit was brought claiming negligence as the result of unreasonable delay in obtaining medical aid. The boy was admitted to the hospital two hours after the accident. In court testimony, a neurosurgeon pointed out that X rays did not reveal the skull fracture and blood clot that caused the death. The physician could not say how much sooner he would have had to have seen the boy in order to save his life.

He further testified that headache and dizziness were "soft" symptoms of brain injury, not of great importance. The crucial signs of brain injury would be loss of consciousness, change in the size of the pupils of the eyes, and weakness in one side of the body. In this situation, the boy did not lose consciousness, the school nurse found the size of the pupils of his eyes to be normal, and there was no evidence of body weakness.

The court found no proof of unreasonable delay in this case, in view of the fact that the boy was sent to a physician by the school within an hour of the accident. The

19. Peck v. Board of Education of City of Mount Vernon, et al., 317 N.Y.S. 2d 919 (1970).

physician admitted the boy to a hospital within two hours of the accident. The court ruled that correct and prompt emergency care procedures had been taken and that there were no grounds for a ruling of negligence in this situation.

Another case which implied that immediate and emergency care services are to be rendered by teachers is important enough to examine. In this situation,[20] a group of girls was playing a game on the school playground during the noon hour. A girl ran her arm through the glass in a door and then jerked her arm back. In so doing, she severed an artery, and serious bleeding resulted. Several girls ran to tell the teacher. Another girl took the injured girl to the nurse's room. When a nurse arrived, she stopped the bleeding by applying direct pressure to the artery. The doctor was called, and he put on a tourniquet. Later that night the girl died as a result of losing so much blood before she was given any emergency care.

The court ruled that negligence was present in this situation. The implication was that emergency care services are to be rendered by teachers, and such care is to be rendered without delay. In this situation, delay had resulted during the time that the nurse was being sought. The teacher should have acted promptly to stop the bleeding, then proceeded to notify the nurse.

It is important that school personnel render only emergency care and not give medical treatment. In a New Jersey litigation,[21] this principle was upheld. During football practice, a boy's shoulder was injured. His parents sued the coaches, alleging that the coaches were negligent in failing to obtain the required medical assistance for the injured player.

---

20. Ogando v. Carquinez Grammar School District of Contra Costa County, et al., 24 Calif. App. 2d 567, 75 P. 2d 641 (1938).
21. Duda, et al. v. Gaines, et al., 12 N.J. Super. 326, 79 A. 2d 695 (1951).

The boy had previously injured the shoulder in an earlier practice session. The boy went to a doctor who put the arm in a sling. The physician told the boy that he could resume football practice in two weeks. During the first practice session after the boy returned, his shoulder was dislocated again. A coach put the dislocated shoulder back in place, put the arm in a sling, and sent the boy home. For several days the boy wore the sling around his home. His parents were aware of the condition during this time.

The parents later sued the coaches, claiming that they were negligent in their actions. The court ruled in favor of the coaches. The decision was based on the concept that there was no pressing necessity for medical treatment in this situation. It was felt that the coaches did render proper emergency care for the boy, and that it was not their responsibility to give medical treatment or to provide for medical treatment. It was the responsibility of the parents to obtain the needed medical treatment.

In administering emergency care, it is very important to know when one's responsibility ends. Usually, it has been assumed that when medical help arrives, a school teacher's or school administrator's responsibility ends. However, in a litigation involving another football injury, a verdict was rendered which seems to indicate that this concept may not be legally acceptable.

In this case,[22] a football player was injured in a practice scrimmage. The coach, suspecting a neck injury, asked the boy to grasp his hand in order to see if he were able to grip. The boy was able to do so. Eight players then carried the injured boy off the field. A physician was present at the scrimmage. There was conflicting testimony as to

22. Welch *v.* Dunsmuir Joint Union High School District, 326 P. 2d 633 (Calif., 1958).

whether the physician had examined the boy before he was removed from the field. Today, the boy is permanently paralyzed as a result of the injuries from this accident. In the litigation that resulted, it was expressed that the damage had not been done by the tackle, as the boy was able to grip with his hand before being moved. The suit held that the damage occurred as he was being moved from the field.

The court ruled that the coach's responsibility did not end when the physician's responsibility began and both the physician and the coach were negligent in having the boy moved from the field. This was a very important precedent set in this case. To date, this decision has not been followed or cited by other courts in similar cases. However, it is a principle of law of which one must be aware.

Even though the courts have ruled that the board of education has the authority to provide emergency care for an injured pupil, the supreme court of appeals in West Virginia[23] handed down a decision that the school board has no authority to pay the attending physician after the emergency has passed. In this case the court recognized the duty of the school board to provide emergency care for an injured pupil. However, the board had no authority to render assistance beyond that required of the emergency itself.

Not only is it necessary to provide reasonable and prudent care for a sick or injured person, but it is also very important that proper, complete, and continuous records be kept of all accidents. This is necessary for even the most seemingly insignificant accident. Consultation with legal authorities will give the administrator direction as to what kinds of records should be kept and for how long they

23. Jarrett v. Goodall, 113 W. Va. 478, 168 S.E. 763 (1933).

should remain on file, in view of local and state rules and regulations.

Minors, in many states, have the power of delayed suit. The power of delayed suit is a person's opportunity, upon reaching adulthood, usually between eighteen and twenty-one years of age, to sue in his own name for an accident which occurred during his school days when he was a minor. Even if the parents sued at the time of the accident and lost, an individual has the power of delayed suit. This exemplifies the need for good accident report forms, signed witness statements, and as complete records as possible.

An example of a delayed suit was a case in New York City.[24] As a fourteen year old boy in the eighth grade in 1950, the plaintiff was required to work in a school stockroom carrying boxes of books. He became sick at the time and experienced pains in the chest. He claimed that six weeks were spent home in bed with myocardial damage to the heart as the result of this experience.

Ten years later in 1960, as an adult, the plaintiff sued the school board, claiming that his present cardiac condition was the result of the experience he had in the stock room. The court supported his case and ordered the school board to pay for damages.

Proper supervisory provisions must be made to protect all concerned from lawsuit regarding matters relating to emergency care. Every school administrator directly responsible for school children should provide, in writing, policies and procedures to be followed in emergency situations involving injury or illness. It is important to develop these policies and procedures in consultation with proper medical and legal authority. Once developed, such written

24. Feuerstein v. Board of Education of the City of New York, 202 N.Y.S. 2d 524 (1960).

regulations must be made known to all school employees—faculty as well as staff. Periodic in-service meetings for the purpose of updating the employees' knowledge and for the purpose of discussing and answering their questions would seem to be extremely valuable.

Summary

It generally has been accepted by the courts that the care expected to be given by an individual in cases of illness or injury is that which an ordinarily prudent person would have exercised under similar circumstances. That degree of responsibility is considered to be greater for school teachers than for the non-teaching individual.

Since the teacher is serving *in loco parentis* with regard to his relationship to school children, it must be assumed that the teacher has a responsibility to render emergency care for a child who becomes sick or injured in the school environment in the same way that the parent would be expected to do if the child were at home. The kind and degree of care to be given has depended upon the circumstances. The circumstances have been weighed very heavily by the courts where emergency care litigation was under consideration.

Only emergency care and not medical treatment is to be rendered by school personnel. Traditionally it has been assumed that the responsibility of the person rendering emergency care ends when the sick or injured is taken to a physician or to other professional help. This concept has been challenged by court opinion and some question might be raised as to its applicability.

In some states, a person, upon reaching the age of majority (or adulthood), has the right of delayed suit. Because of this, it is very important that proper records be kept of all reportable accident situations within the school.

All of these concepts are important to the school personnel in light of the definitions of liability and of negligence. With the gradually changing attitude toward immunity of governmental agencies by courts and state legislatures, the school administrator and teacher need to take a very close look at those rules and regulations of their own schools relating to emergency care procedures.

6
Immunization and Vaccination

State statutes, state board of health regulations, and school district rules and regulations requiring vaccination and immunization of pupils have led to more litigations than any other aspect of the school health services program. Normally, two important questions have arisen with respect to requiring vaccinations and immunizations of children in the public schools: 1) Are state statutes and school board or board of health regulations legal which make vaccination a condition for attendance? 2) Can the schools compel vaccination or exclusion from school as a means of controlling or preventing the spread of disease during an epidemic or suspected period of emergency involving the particular disease?

One other question came before the courts in the latter years of the nineteenth century and in the early years of the twentieth century. The question raised in objection to vaccination requirements asked whether vaccination could actually prevent smallpox. These cases claimed that vaccination was not a preventive of smallpox. It often was felt that the practice of vaccination actually was harmful. As such, it was believed by many to be injurious to the child rather than beneficial. In raising such an objection, people believed that vaccination had nothing to do with the eradication of smallpox.

An example of opposition to immunization was a case in 1919 in North Dakota[1] in which a Supreme Court judge issued a very strong warning to the advocates of vaccination as a preventive measure against smallpox. In his statement, the judge said:

> The proper safeguard is by sanitation. The chances are that within a generation vaccination will cease to exist. It will go the way of inoculation, bleeding, purging, and salvation. The vaccinators must learn to live without sowing the seeds of death and disease.

As recently as 1940, a court in Pennsylvania heard testimony that vaccination for smallpox "is often responsible for appendicitis, syphilis, sleeping sickness, infantile paralysis, tetanus and other harmful results and in many cases, death."[2] This testimony was refuted in court by the Director of the Bureau of Health and Sanitation of the Pennsylvania State Department of Health. In the intervening years, this question has not arisen in courts of law. Today, it is a scientific fact, quite universally accepted, that vaccination does prevent smallpox.

Vaccination certificates and immunization reports are often required by state statute, board of health regulations, or school district rules and regulations as a prerequisite

---

1. Rhea *v.* Board of Education of Devils Lake Special School District, 171 N.W. 108 (N.D., 1919).
2. Marsh, In re., 14 A. 2d 370 (Pa., 1940).

for enrollment into school. These requirements have been challenged quite frequently in the courts. The courts have handed down decisions which have established the principle that passing a law requiring vaccination of school children, as a condition for their being admitted to the public school, is legal and not in violation of the constitutional rights of children. Many of the legal precedents are rather dated; however, it is still important for the school administrator to know what decisions have been rendered.

Common Law Principles

The United States Supreme Court, in the case of Jacobson *v.* the Commonwealth of Massachusetts,[3] held that the enactment of a statute requiring compulsory vaccination for the protection of the public against the spread of smallpox was legal. It felt that such statutes do not deprive an individual of his constitutional guarantees of personal and religious liberty. It was stated by the Supreme Court:

But the liberty secured by the Constitution of the United States to every person within its jurisdiction does not import an absolute right in each person to be, at all times and in all circumstances, wholly freed from restraint . . . This court has more than once recognized it as a fundamental principle that 'persons and property are subjected to all kinds of restraints and burdens, in order to secure the general comfort, health, and prosperity of the State.'

In further developing the basic principle for its decision, the Supreme Court said:

---

3. Jacobson *v.* Commonwealth of Massachusetts, 197 U.S. 11, 255 S. Ct. 358 (1905).

Upon the principle of self-defense, of paramount necessity, a community has the right to protect itself against an epidemic of disease which threatens the safety of its members.

This ruling by the United States Supreme Court has been a very important point of law. The principle established in this case has been extensively followed by other courts in support of similar decisions. It also has an implication for any future cases involving vaccination, immunization, or the teaching of health-related subjects in the school curriculum.

Such findings by the courts have been based on the concept that statutes requiring vaccination and immunization of school children are a valid exercise of the police power of the state. The local school district is an agent of the state, and by requiring vaccination and immunization of school children, it is fulfilling, in part, its police powers intended to protect others in the community.

The Supreme Court of New Hampshire[4] stated that it is a reasonable measure for the protection of the health of the public when referring to a statute requiring vaccination for admittance to school.

If a statute exists requiring the vaccination of pupils as a requirement for admittance to school, the statute must be considered to be mandatory unless it clearly is stated as being of a permissive nature. This viewpoint was supported by the California Court of Appeals[5] which rendered an opinion regarding a state of California statute requiring vaccination. The court stated:

4. State v. Drew, 192 A. 629 (N.H., 1937).
5. State Board of Health v. Board of Trustees of Watsonville School Dist. of Santa Cruz County, et al., 110 P. 138 (Calif., 1910).

The statute is not directory, but mandatory. . . . It is the plain duty of the trustees, and they are directed by the express terms of the statute, to exclude from the public schools any child or person who has not been vaccinated. . . . The duty devolves upon defendants by virtue of their office to exclude such children. They must obey and not question the law.

School boards and school administrators have no choice but to comply with the statutes, even though some people may bring suit, as has been done in numerous instances.

The Supreme Court of Arkansas upheld a statute requiring vaccination of school children, declaring that such a health regulation has the force and effect of law.[6] An earlier case in the same state found the Arkansas Supreme Court supporting a lower court decision[7] when it ruled that unless a state statute gives the parents the right, no legal right was available for parents to prevent vaccination of their children. In this case, the court ruled that the children must submit to vaccination before they could be admitted to school. The parents refused to permit their children to be vaccinated because of personal religious beliefs. The court held that the right to have religious freedom does not permit the right to refuse vaccination. The principle set forth was that a person's right to religious freedom ceases where it transgresses upon the rights of others. Refusing to be vaccinated infringes upon the rights of another person to have freedom from communicable disease. The Arkansas Supreme Court summarized its conclusions in this manner:

6. Mannis v. State ex rel. DeWitt School District #1, 398 S.W. 2d 206 (Ark., 1966).
7. Cude v. State, 377 S.W. 2d 816 (Ark., 1964).

The school administrative authorities of the State of Arkansas have adopted a regulation requiring vaccination . . . There is no question about the validity of this regulation . . . The Constitution of Arkansas provides . . . that anyone has the right to worship God in the manner of his own choice, but it does not mean that he can engage in religious practices inconsistent with the peace, safety and health of the inhabitants of the State, and it does not mean that parents, on religious grounds, have the right to deny their children an education.

In Ohio,[8] a law was passed requiring immunization against polio, smallpox, pertussis, and tetanus as a requirement for entrance to school. Suit was brought against the school board of Covington, Ohio, challenging this law. The court ruled that a child did not have the right to enter school without the immunizations. The court further stated that the school board had the authority to make and enforce rules and regulations, seeing that all children were immunized. The upholding of statutory provisions requiring immunization for polio, smallpox, and measles of all school children was supported as recently as 1969 in litigation in New York.[9]

Various decisions have been rendered which suggest that the refusal of parents to have their children vaccinated before the child may be admitted to school amounts to a transgression of the rights of others. At least two courts have ruled that the exclusion of a child from school because he had not been vaccinated did not excuse the parent from fulfilling his responsibility in seeing that the child met the requirement of compulsory attendance at

8. State *ex rel.* Mack *v.* Board of Education of Covington, 204 N.E. 2d 86 (Ohio, 1963).
9. McCartney, *et al. v.* Austin, *et al.,* 298 N.Y.S. 2d 26 (1969).

school. The parent can be found guilty of and be convicted for not sending the child to school.[10]

It also has been ruled in several cases that refusal to comply with health regulations requiring vaccinations and immunizations was sufficient evidence upon which to base a finding of child neglect against the parents. In a case in New York,[11] the parents did not permit the children to be immunized for polio, in spite of a public health law which prohibited children from attending school unless they had a polio immunization. The children were considered to be "neglected children" by the family court, based on an opinion that the children were not being provided with an education.

In Pennsylvania,[12] a boy's father refused to have his son vaccinated for smallpox. The child was refused admission to school and sent home because he failed to produce evidence that he had been vaccinated for or that he had previously had smallpox. For nearly six weeks, the student came to school, but was refused admission each time. For approximately two years the child did not attend school. His father was convicted several times and imprisoned for violating the compulsory school attendance laws. A hearing resulted, and the child was found to be neglected as a result of his father's not obeying the compulsory school attendance laws and seeing that his son was provided with an education. As a result, the child was ordered to be committed to the care of the local welfare services until his father would abide by the compulsory school attendance laws. The father appealed the decision which gave the

10. Commonwealth v. Green, 268 Mass. 585, 168 N.E. 101 (1929). State v. Drew, 192 A. 629 (N.H., 1937).
11. Elwell, In re., 284 N.Y.S. 2d 924 (1967).
12. Marsh, In re., 140 Pa. Super. 472, 14 A. 2d 368 (1940).

county welfare services custody of the boy. However, the action was upheld by the superior court of Pennsylvania, based on the finding that the father was neglectful in relationship to the care and welfare of his son.

Not only have the courts supported decisions requiring that school children be immunized against various diseases, but also the same rulings regarding teachers have been upheld by the courts. In the case of Lyndall v. the High School Committee in Pennsylvania,[13] a teacher was suspended from her teaching position because she did not comply with a school board resolution requiring vaccination of teachers against smallpox. The teacher sought an injunction against this suspension. The injunction was denied, and the court rendered the opinion that teachers and other school employees could be required to submit to vaccination against smallpox. It would be reasonable to expect teachers and school personnel to abide by the same rulings and regulations required of students for the protection of the health and welfare of the public within the framework of the schools.

Where statutory provision, health department regulations, or school board rules and regulations require vaccination and immunization before admittance to school is permitted, it should be evident that such requirements are to be fulfilled. However, there are schools where no such regulations are available for rendering direction to the school administrator. What is to be the policy in these situations when an epidemic condition or an abnormal situation arises?

In time of possible epidemics or emergency situations involving a specific disease, the courts have ruled that admission to the public schools can be restricted to those children who have been vaccinated. Those who have not

13. Lyndall v. High School Committee, 19 Pa. Super. Ct. 232 (1901).

been vaccinated can be prevented from attending school during the period of suspected epidemic or emergency. One of the earliest cases raising the question of attendance at school in time of epidemic conditions was the case of Duffield v. the Williamsport School District in 1894.[14] In this case, a child who had not been vaccinated against smallpox was not permitted to come to school. The decision was based on a local board of health ruling that only vaccinated children be permitted to attend school. The ruling had been made because smallpox was at that time present in the town and had been in epidemic proportions in other nearby communities. It was pointed out in court that at no time was the child forced to submit to vaccination; he just could not go to school during the epidemic danger period. The court found that this regulation was a reasonable ruling, based on the fact that it benefited the general public and protected the health of others. The decision and opinion rendered in this case has since been cited extensively in some twenty-two additional states and in numerous other similar litigations.

Not just state health departments may require students to be vaccinated, but local and city health departments may also make regulations governing student attendance at school in time of epidemic or emergency. As early as 1900, the Indiana Supreme Court handed down a ruling upholding the right of a local board of health to require that school children be vaccinated for smallpox or else they not be permitted to attend school during a period of smallpox epidemic.[15] In this case, a boy was prohibited from attending school because he had not been vaccinated

14. Duffield v. School District of City of Williamsport, 162 Pa. 476, 29 A. 742 (1894).
15. Blue v. Beach, et al., 56 N.E. 89 (Ind., 1900).

against smallpox. The state board of health had adopted a rule which made it necessary that children be vaccinated for smallpox, when there was danger of an epidemic, before the child would be admitted to school. The local board of health was given power to enforce such a requirement. The school board in Terre Haute was directed by the local board of health not to allow any person to attend school unless he had been vaccinated. There were no state statutes making vaccination compulsory for school attendance. Therefore, the suit questioned the legality of the regulation made by the board of health. The Indiana Supreme Court ruled that the school board was justified in excluding the student from school during the period of emergency or danger of smallpox. This ruling held, even though the child was not found to have smallpox. The court pointed out that children may be expelled from school for violating certain rules of school discipline. In a judge's concurring opinion, it was stated:

> If expulsion can result from the violation of a rule, the object of which is to promote the morals of the scholars, and the efficiency of the school in general, certainly one which is intended and calculated to promote the health of the scholars ought to be sustained.

Through the years, this decision has been referred to numerous times in litigations involving vaccination and immunization requirements in the schools. The principles of law established in this case have been cited in over one hundred other cases in support of decisions reached regarding the requirement that students be vaccinated and immunized against a variety of diseases.

Several years later in a similar case in Indiana,[16] a ruling

---

16. Vonnegut v. Baum, 188 N.E. 677 (Ind., 1934).

was given that a *city* board of health could exclude children from school who had not been vaccinated, upon the determination of an emergency or danger of a smallpox epidemic. This case was similar to the Blue *v.* Beach case. A municipal board of health ruling was passed. This ruling required that all pupils must be vaccinated for smallpox or otherwise be excluded from school. In the opinion of the health department authorities, there was danger of a smallpox epidemic. The incidences of the disease were increasing, and it was felt that a public health emergency existed. The authority of the municipal board of health to issue such a ruling was challenged in court. The court held that the resolution of the city board of health was authorized and legal. In rendering the decision, the court stated that such a resolution "prevents children who have not been vaccinated from attending school during an emergency in which they might transmit the disease to other school children or carry it from other school children back to their homes."

The legal principle that the local board of health may declare a state of emergency and require all pupils to be vaccinated before admittance to school was upheld in a court decision in Michigan.[17] However, a very important question was raised by one of the dissenting justices. The dissenting question asked how many cases of a particular disease must be present in order to constitute an epidemic condition.

There was smallpox in Lansing during the winter of 1922-1923. The local board of health passed a resolution requiring that all children, teachers, and other school personnel who had not been vaccinated should be excluded

17. People *ex rel.* Hill *v.* Board of Education of City of Lansing, *et al.*, 224 Mich. 388, 195 N.W. 95 (1923).

from the public schools. The local board of health declared that epidemic conditions were present. The school board challenged this assertion. Their challenge presented the fact that there were only seventeen reported cases of smallpox in a school population of approximately eleven thousand. It seemed to the school district that this number of cases did not warrant epidemic conditions. No specific answer was given to their question. However, the court did uphold the board of health's resolution. This seems to indicate that the declaration of an emergency or epidemic condition is solely up to the discretion of the board of health authorities. The criteria which the board of health wishes to use in determining if conditions are of an epidemic proportion are left to the decision of the board.

Even though the Lansing school board objected to the board of health ruling, the court proceeded to support the fact that the authority of the board of health was legal in situations of potential epidemic conditions. The principle was established that the school board must enforce rulings of the board of health in times of an emergency, even if it disagrees with the regulation.

In the absence of a potential epidemic, several courts have upheld the ruling that the *local* authorities could not require a vaccination or immunization as a condition for school admission if no statutory or state health department regulations were available.

This principle of law was affirmed by the North Dakota Supreme Court in 1919.[18] There was no statute requiring vaccination in North Dakota at that time. The court held that the local board of health was not authorized to issue a regulation prohibiting children from attending public

18. Rhea *v.* Board of Education of Devils Lake Special School District, 41 N.D. 449, 171 N.W. 103 (1919).

schools except when there was an epidemic condition present.

In a similar case in Wisconsin,[19] the same principle of law was upheld. A rule by the state board of health, stating that no one could attend school without presenting evidence that he had been vaccinated against smallpox when there was no epidemic, was judged to be void by the Wisconsin Supreme Court. There was no statute requiring vaccination at that time; therefore, unless an epidemic was present throughout the state, no such regulation was legal.

A school board may require that a specific method of vaccination be employed. In the case of Allen v. Ingalls,[20] a child was vaccinated for smallpox by a physician of the homeopathic school of medicine. The homeopathic method of vaccination involved an internal procedure of vaccination. Medicine in powder form was administered orally.

The child brought to school a certificate stating that he had been vaccinated by this method. The school board refused to accept this certificate of vaccination, claiming that it did not meet the requirements of the law. The law required that the vaccine be of the bovine virus and must be injected through the skin. The homeopathic procedure did not satisfy this requirement. For this reason, the child was denied the right to attend school. The court upheld the position of the school board regulation in this case. It was ruled that the school district could stipulate what method of vaccination must be used in fulfilling the requirement for vaccination.

The same opinion was rendered by the Court of Civil Appeals of Texas.[21] In this case, a school requirement that

---

19. State ex. rel. Adams v. Burdge, et al., 70 N.W. 347 (Wisc., 1897).
20. Allen et al. v. Ingalls, et al., 182 Ark. 991, 33 S.W. 2d 1099 (1930).
21. Abney v. Fox, et al., 250 S.W. 210 (Tex., 1923).

smallpox vaccination be by scarification and injection of cowpox was upheld by the court. The regulation requiring this method of vaccination rather than the taking of medicine internally was ruled legally acceptable. Even if it could have been proven that the internal method was effective, the school board regulation requiring a specific method was permissible.

It is important to note that one of the judges presented a very strong dissenting opinion regarding the ruling in this case. The basis for his dissent was stated as follows:

> The homeopathic treatment administered . . . is equally as effective as a preventative of smallpox as is vaccination by scarification. . . . No school board or city or town council, under its general authority to protect the public health, has the implied authority to require anyone to be vaccinated in any manner, unless the same appears to be reasonably necessary to prevent such person from taking the smallpox, and thereby communicate it to others.

The courts also have ruled that the school board may require that a certificate of evidence of vaccination must be shown before the child can enter school,[22] and that the school board may regulate the form of certificate to be used.[23]

The question of infringement on religious freedom often has arisen as to whether a student must submit to vaccination and immunization requirements prior to enrolling in school. The courts have stood on the principle that the United States Constitution, in establishing the principle of religious freedom, did not do so at the risk of and so as

22. Auten *v.* Board of Directors of Special School District of Little Rock, 83 Ark. 431, 104 S.W. 130 (1907). State *ex rel.* Horne *v.* Beil, *et al.*, 60 N.E. 672 (Ind., 1901).
23. Lee *v.* Marsh, 230 Pa. 351, 79 A. 564 (1911).

to endanger the safety, health, and welfare of an individual. This subject will be dealt with in detail in the following chapter.

Statutory Provisions

State statutory provision relating to vaccination and immunization requirements usually either 1) identify the specific diseases for which a child must be immunized or 2) authorize the state health department to make the requirements and regulations it feels necessary for the protection of the general public. Several states specify that no child is to be admitted to school with an infectious disease. The state department of health, in these cases, is given the responsibility for determining specific regulations. This might mean establishment of regulations for vaccination and immunization, regulations specifying when a child is to be admitted or refused admittance to school, or a number of other possible provisions. About one-half of the states have no statutory provision regarding vaccination and immunization requirements. However, in these states, state and local boards of education often establish their own regulations.

The disease conditions for which a statutory requirement is most commonly available are smallpox, tetanus, diphtheria, pertussis, and polio. In the past couple of years, rubeola and rubella (measles and German measles, respectively) have been added by some state legislatures.

TABLE 5 *States Where Statutory Provision Authorizes the State Department of Health to Establish Regulations Regarding Vaccination and Immunization*

Alaska	Missouri
California	Nebraska

Georgia
Maryland
Massachusetts

New Mexico
Rhode Island
Tennessee

TABLE 6 *Diseases for Which Vaccination and Immunization Are Required by State Statute*

Arkansas: polio, diphtheria, tetanus, pertussis, rubeola
California: smallpox
Connecticut: smallpox, measles, polio
Illinois: measles, smallpox, tetanus, diphtheria, polio, pertussis
Indiana: smallpox, tetanus, diphtheria, polio, pertussis
Kansas: rubeola, smallpox, tetanus, diphtheria, polio, pertussis, rubella
Kentucky: measles, smallpox, tetanus, diphtheria, polio
Louisiana: measles, smallpox, tetanus, diphtheria, polio, pertussis
Maryland: smallpox
Massachusetts: measles, smallpox, tetanus, diphtheria, polio, pertussis
New Hampshire: smallpox
New Jersey: diphtheria, polio, measles
North Carolina: polio
Ohio: polio, smallpox, diphtheria, pertussis, tetanus, rubella, rubeola
Oklahoma: polio, smallpox, diphtheria, pertussis, tetanus, rubeola
Pennsylvania: smallpox
Virginia: smallpox
West Virginia: smallpox, diphtheria, polio, measles, tetanus, pertussis

One state (North Dakota) has a statute which states that no form of vaccination shall be required as a prerequisite for admission to school. Needless to say, this is a very unusual provision.

Statutory regulations in the various states almost always include a provision exempting children whose parents oppose on religious grounds having their children vaccinated or immunized. Usually the procedure to be followed involves the child's parents or guardian writing a letter to the school authorities requesting exemption from the requirement because of religious beliefs. Exemption is also provided for those children who because of health and/or medical reasons cannot be immunized.

Specific local board of education regulations, where no statutory provisions are available, are too numerous for inclusion in this chapter. However, they basically follow the same guidelines as presented in this section with regard to statutory provisions.

Summary

Litigation has been very extensive with respect to rules and regulations concerning vaccination and immunization procedures. Overwhelmingly, court precedent has supported statutory requirements, health department regulations, and school board rules and regulations providing for vaccination and immunization of school children. Court opinion supporting vaccination and immunization requirements is based on the concept that such provisions are a valid exercise of the police power of the state for the protection of the health of the public.

Refusal to comply with health regulations requiring vaccination and immunization has been found to be sufficient evidence upon which to base a finding of child neglect against the parents.

Where no statutory provision is available, the courts have ruled that a child who has not been vaccinated or immunized may be excluded from school during an epidemic condition. State, county, and local health departments may make and enforce rulings of this nature when epidemic conditions warrant such action.

Not only may children be excluded from school who lack required vaccination and immunization procedures, but teachers also may be required to show proof of having been vaccinated and immunized.

Statutory provisions are available in a majority of the

states. State statutory provisions relating to vaccination and immunization requirements usually either 1) identify the specific diseases for which a child must be immunized or 2) authorize the state health department to make the requirements and regulations it feels necessary for the protection of the general public. Where no statutory provision is available and no health department regulations give direction, local board of education regulations are usually available giving direction to the school administrator as to which vaccinations and immunizations are necessary before a child may attend school.

The question of infringement on religious freedom has often been raised in challenging regulations requiring vaccination and immunization. Court precedent has suggested that such requirements are not an infringement of one's religious freedom. This topic will be developed more completely in the next chapter. States having statutory requirements will usually include a provision exempting those who oppose on religious grounds from having to submit to the vaccination and immunization regulations.

7

Religious Conflicts and the School Health Program

The question of infringement on religious freedom often has arisen in relation to various aspects of the school health program. School districts' requiring of medical examinations for enrollment in school, requiring of certain immunization procedures, and the teaching of health concepts and information in the classroom have presented problems for people of several religious beliefs. Usually a state statute or school district ruling and regulation will make provision for exempting children, whose parents object to such procedures, on religious grounds. The provision usually will require a parental signed statement expressing the family's objections to certain health services or instruction as a basis for such exemption of the child.

Where there are no provisions made, legal precedent must be understood. The courts have stood on the principle that the United States Constitution, in establishing the principle of religious freedom, did not do so at the risk of and so as to endanger the safety, health, and well-being of an individual. This principle of law was affirmed in a Kentucky case[1] where the court upheld certain state statutes, stating that the federal constitution does not preclude a state from passing a law prohibiting the practice of some religious rite which endangers the health or safety of the public. It was not the purpose of the United States Constitution, according to this court, to permit under the guise of religious freedom those activities which would endanger or harm another person.

Various other legal opinions have resulted from litigation concerning this subject. In a New York case, the court stated that "the practice of one's religion must be exercised in the light of the general public welfare, and cannot conflict with the public welfare. Acts which are not worship are not necessarily guaranteed."[2] In this case, the court found that a state statute requiring immunization of school children against polio as a prerequisite for their admission to school was legal and did not infringe upon one's rights or privileges guaranteed under the United States Constitution.

In the case of Wright v. DeWitt School District,[3] the parents and their children were members of a church which did not permit immunization of its members. The parents claimed that a state health regulation requiring a smallpox vaccination as a prerequisite to attend school was in violation of their religious freedom. The court ruled that the regulation was reasonable and stated that "freedom to act according to their religious beliefs is subject to a reasonable regulation for the benefit of society as a whole."

1. Lawson, et al. v. Commonwealth, 291 Ky. 437, 164 S.W. 2d 972 (1942).
2. Elwell, In re., 284 N.Y.S. 2d 930 (1967).
3. Wright v. DeWitt School Dist. No. 1 of Arkansas County, 385 S.W. 2d 644 (Ark., 1965).

If an individual objects to health requirements because of personal religious beliefs, but is a member of a religious organization that does not include such prohibition as part of the dogma of that faith, what is to be the position of the school administration? A court in North Carolina[4] ruled that a father did not have to prove that the religious organization of which he was a member prohibited immunization in order to warrant statutory exemption. The father was a member of a religious fellowship group that did not forbid immunization. However, they believed that faith in God kept a person in good health and, as individuals, the members could object to immunization procedures. Therefore, the parents in this case were not required to have their children immunized. Personal objection based upon religious beliefs and not membership in a particular church was the determining consideration.

The same basic concept was upheld in a case in the state of New Jersey.[5] In this situation, the Supreme Court of New Jersey ruled that membership in some specific religious group, *i.e.*, the Christian Science faith, could not be required as a condition for exemption from vaccination. A student wishing to enroll at Rutgers University refused to undergo a physical examination and certain required immunizations as prerequisites for admittance into the school. This student also refused to sign a statement indicating that he was a member of the Christian Science faith or of any other sect or religion. He based his opposition to the requirement on personal religious grounds, believing that God would keep him healthy, not membership in some specific faith.

The court ruled in favor of the student. It was the

4. State *v.* Miday, 140 S.E. 2d 325 (N.C., 1966).
5. Kolbeck *v.* Kramer, 84 N.J. Super. 569, 202 A. 2d 889 (1964).

opinion of the court that an individual did not have to declare membership in a specific group in order to be exempted from the requirement. The school was directed to enroll the student without his undergoing the physical examinations and immunizations. The court stated that "while it is true that all Christian Scientists may be entitled to an exemption, all those who are entitled to exemptions need not be Christian Scientists."

In an earlier case in New Jersey,[6] a woman of the Christian Science faith sponsored three children from Greece for a twelve-month stay in the United States. Upon enrolling these children in school, she came into conflict with a New Jersey statute requiring diphtheria immunizations. The basis for her objection was that such immunizations were against her personal religious beliefs. The children were not of the Christian Science faith, but were Greek Orthodox.

The court ruled against the woman and, among other supporting court cases in expressing their opinion, quoted from Mary Baker Eddy, the founder of the Christian Science Church, as follows:

> Rather than quarrel over vaccination, I recommend, if the law demand, that an individual submit to this process, that he obey the law, and then appeal to the gospel to save him from bad physical results. . . . I believe in obeying the laws of the land.[7]

A statutory provision in New York requiring polio, smallpox, and measles immunization has been challenged in court. This statute exempts individuals from the basic re-

---

6. Board of Education of Mountain Lakes *v.* Maas, 152 A. 2d 394 (N.J., 1959).
7. *Ibid.,* pp. 407–408.

quirements for immunization who are members of recognized religious groups that do not permit such practices. In this case,[8] the family was of the Roman Catholic religion. The Roman Catholic Church does not have any teachings prohibiting health examinations, immunizations, or instruction concerning similar health matters. However, the family brought litigation, claiming that the law was unconstitutional. The basis for claiming that the statutory provision was unconstitutional was based on the grounds that it was discriminatory. The court ruled that this provision, which required all students to have polio, smallpox, and measles immunizations, was constitutional. The provision for exemption of certain persons for religious beliefs did not make the requirement void.

Summary

The weight of law seems to support the principle that any action which is of a nature dangerous to the health and welfare of others cannot be condoned under the principle of religious freedom. Nevertheless, statutory legislation should make provision for consideration of the religious beliefs of people regarding health and medical care. It is important to be aware of the state statutory provisions, as well as common law principles, when establishing rules and regulations regarding immunization, requirements for medical examinations of school children, in planning the health education instructional program, and in establishing other policies relating to the various phases and programs of the school health program.

---

8. McCartney, *et al. v.* Austin, *et al.*, 298 N.Y.S. 2d 26 (1969).

8
Healthful School Environment

General Considerations

The legal basis for providing a healthful school environment rests on the fact that education is compulsory in the United States. The child legally is required to be sent to school during certain years of his life. For this reason, it must be assumed that the child will be coming to an environment which is safe and is conducive to good health. Because of this, each state has specific regulations governing location of the school, regulations for proper sanitation, for safe and clean water supply and various other health related provisions. It is the responsibility of the school administrator to be familiar with the regulations governing his school district. Legal responsibility for proper environmental procedures in the schools often rests with the particular state board of health. The schools must see that health department regulations are met and upheld.

The courts have held that the school environment or school building consists of more than the physical edifice

111

within which actual class instruction takes place. The general principle followed by the courts in rendering a decision regarding health and safety within a school has been that a school building is a facility designed to be used in carrying out any part of the instructional program authorized by the school board. Basing opinions upon this principle, swimming pool facilities were considered a part of the school building facility in a case in Oregon.[1] In Iowa,[2] a football field was considered part of the school "building."

It is the obligation of the school board to provide a safe and healthy school environment for the children. The health and the physical condition of students while at school are influenced by the environmental conditions of the school.

As early as 1887, the Indiana Supreme Court expressed an opinion that rules and regulations of the school must give special attention to the health, comfort, and physical condition of the students. Rules and regulations which may be dangerous to the pupils' health and well-being must not be made by school authorities. A widely accepted principle of law is that the schools have the power to make reasonable rules and regulations for the operation of the school. In establishing rules and regulations, the school district must not only develop rules that are for the good of the school, but, also, considerations must be given to the health, comfort, and the effect of the environment on the physical condition of students.

In the 1887 Indiana case,[3] testimony pointed out that

1. School Board of School District No. U2-20 JT., Multnomah County v. Fanning, 377 P. 2d 4 (Ore., 1962).
2. City of Bloomfield v. Davis County Community School District, 119 N.W. 2d 909 (Iowa, 1963).
3. Fertich v. Michener, 111 Ind. 472, 11 N.E. 605 (1887).

a teacher had the policy of locking the doors during the opening exercises which were conducted at the start of each school day. On one particular winter day, a student arrived at school late. The opening exercises had begun, and the doors were locked. The temperature was eighteen degrees below zero, and the ground was covered with snow. Upon finding the school doors locked, the student returned home, and in the process her feet became frozen.

The court was of the opinion that the action by the teacher, locking the school doors during opening exercises, was an acceptable practice when the weather was moderate. However, in cold weather this practice was dangerous to the health of the students, and the practice of locking the doors was an unreasonable act.

This same principle, that the school district is responsible for providing a safe and healthy school environment for the children, was emphasized in a court case in New York.[4] In this situation, a boy, while running on the school ground at noon, tripped over a wire strung about two to three inches from the ground and fell on a metal post. No one knew who placed the wire on the school grounds. The court ruled that under New York statute the school board was obligated to provide safe and adequate school grounds, buildings, and equipment. This principle has been generally accepted throughout the United States.

Another example of this principle is illustrated in the case of Molinari v. Boston.[5] A student was injured by a dangerously exposed steam radiator and pipes in a schoolroom. The court held that the city of Boston could not be held liable for negligence because of the common law

4. Popow v. Central School Dist. No. 1, et al., 251 App. Div. 906, 297 N.Y.S. 205 (1937).
5. Molinari v. The City of Boston, 130 N.E. 2d 925 (Mass., 1955).

doctrine of governmental immunity. However, the opinion was expressed that it was the duty of the school board to provide and maintain a school environment conducive to good health and the welfare of all the students.

Hazards within the school environment have been a frequent source of litigation. In Oregon,[6] suit was brought against the school district in which it was alleged that the school failed to keep a sidewalk on the school premises in a reasonably safe condition. The sidewalk was made of wood and several of the boards of the walk were loose and rotted, with rusty nails protruding above the planks. A student fell on the walk and one of the rusty nails penetrated his knee. The fall resulted in permanent injury to the student.

This situation was taken to court and the school board was charged with negligence in the operation of a safe school environment. The court held that the school district was not liable because the construction and maintenance of a sidewalk on school grounds were governmental functions. As such, the school was free from liability for tort based on the common law doctrine of governmental immunity. Even though the charges against the school district were not upheld by the court, this case is important because it pointed out a potentially hazardous condition in the school environment which was a cause of litigation.

Not only must safe facilities be provided, but the condition and maintenance of these facilities is important. A major factor in lawsuits involving dangerous conditions within the school environment is the determination as to whether or not the school authorities were aware of the condition. The school authorities must not only be aware

6. Lovell v. School District No. 13, Coos County, 143 P. 2d 236 (Ore., 1943).

of any potentially hazardous condition, but they must also proceed to take steps to improve such dangerous environmental conditions.

This legal principle can be seen very clearly in a California case.[7] A sixteen year old boy slipped on a ramp at school and broke his leg. The carpet covering the ramp had worn away in spots. As a result, the ramp had become slippery. Other students also had fallen at this same location. It was pointed out in the court hearing that the school authorities knew of the condition of the ramp. Since no action had been taken to correct this condition, it was the ruling of the court that the school authorities were negligent. The ruling was based on the fact that the school authorities knew of the condition of the ramp but failed to do anything about it.

Another example in which the school authorities failed to correct a potentially dangerous condition occurred in New York.[8] A child was injured while playing on the fire escape at the school. The door leading to the fire escape was defective and the school authorities had been notified of this danger. No attempt had been made to repair the defective door. This lack of action was found to be an act of negligence on the part of the school district. It would appear that every employee of the school district assumes some responsibility for the conditions of the environment within which each child spends a good part of the school day.

Injury resulting from a fall on a wet floor was the source of another litigation recently in New York.[9] A fifteen-year-

---

7. Andre, *et al.* *v.* Allyn, *et al.*, 190 P. 2d 949 (Calif., 1948).
8. Miller *v.* Board of Education, Union Free School, Dist. No. 1, of Town of Albion, *et al.*, 291 N.Y. 25, 50 N.E. 2d 529 (1943).
9. Young *v.* City of New York, *et al.*, 307 N.Y.S. 2d 576 (1970).

old boy slipped on a wet terrazzo floor in the vestibule of the school on a rainy day. Expert testimony stated that such floors are slippery when wet. The idea was expressed that rubber mats should be used on such floors. At the particular entrance where the student fell there was no rubber mat. Failure to provide the mats on such a surface was felt by the plaintiff to be an act of negligence. It was the opinion of the Supreme Court, Appellate Division, in New York that the question of negligence was to be decided by a jury.

The importance of maintaining a safe exit and a well-lighted hallway and stairway is illustrated in another case in New York.[10] A student left the auditorium which was located on the second floor of the building. It was after dark, and there was no light in the hallway or on the stairways. The student had to "feel" her way through the darkened area. However, the handrail, which she was using to guide her down the stairs, ended three steps from the landing. As a result the girl fell and was injured. Suit resulted from this incident. The court ruled that the school district was negligent in not providing a safe school environment. The failure to provide light on the stairway in the school building, as well as the faulty handrail, was considered an act of negligence.

Not only must the school district provide a safe school environment, but that environment must also not be detrimental to the health of the school children. The fact that the school board is responsible for maintaining a healthful school environment was emphasized in a case that took place in Minnesota.[11] In this situation, a teacher had to

10. Hovey v. State, 261 App. Div. 759, 27 N.Y.S. 2d 195 (1941).
11. Bang v. Independent School Dist. No. 27 of St. Louis County, 225 N.W. 449 (Minn., 1929).

retire from teaching because she had tuberculosis. The replacement teacher taught for six weeks. About four months later this individual developed tuberculosis. She brought suit against the school district. Her claim was that the school district made no effort to clean or disinfect the school building after the original teacher found it necessary to quit because of tuberculosis. It was held that the school board did not attempt to protect the successor to the vacated teaching position by maintaining a healthful school environment. The question of whether the plaintiff became infected at school was not raised in this case. The only matter of concern to which the court addressed itself was whether the school district had fulfilled its responsibility of maintaining a healthful school environment.

It is interesting to note that the school district was not found liable for tort. This finding was based on the application of the doctrine of governmental immunity. However, the school district was negligent in its failure to maintain a healthy school environment. The school board had failed to take the proper precautions of cleansing and disinfecting the school rooms.

Not only must state rulings and regulations be known and followed, but, also, local ordinances pertaining to the health and safety standards of public school facilities have been upheld by court decisions. In Illinois,[12] the office of the state superintendent of public instruction issued a publication which included *minimum* requirements for school building specifications. The school board of Rockford, Illinois, challenged the constitutionality of such a statute and requested relief from enforcement of the law in its city schools. The Rockford board of education pointed out that

---

12. Board of Education of the City of Rockford v. Page, et al., 33 Ill. 2d 372, 211 N.E. 2d 361 (1965).

their schools already complied with standards established by the National Fire Prevention Code, local building electrical and plumbing codes, State Department of Public Health laws, and various other recommended standards. It was estimated that to meet the new specifications put forth by the state department of public instruction, it would cost the school district $60,000 for the purpose of surveying all local school facilities and $1 million to comply with all of the specifications.

The Illinois Supreme Court ruled that the right to make this code was legal. Its publication was found to be a proper delegation of administrative authority by the state legislature to the state superintendent for the purpose of protecting the health and welfare of the students. However, the court felt that these standards were not to be considered as being minimum standards. It was pointed out that the standards appeared to be of a *maximum* nature and as such tended to strike down all local ordinances pertaining to health and safety standards of public schools. These specific standards, as published by the state department of instruction, were ruled by the Supreme Court of Illinois to be invalid. It was felt that the already existing local codes were of a higher standard than the proposed state code. The court summarized its position by stating that no state recommendation is to eliminate local codes and ordinances pertaining to the health and safety standards for school buildings.

Oftentimes, seemingly harmless objects within the classroom can be a potential source of danger. This can be illustrated from a case in New York.[13] In this situation, an eleven-year-old child, after opening two windows with a

13. Applebaum *v.* Board of Education of City of New York, 297 N.Y. 762, 77 N.E. 2d 785 (1948).

window pole, carried the pole across the classroom towards the door. In the process of proceeding across the room, the pole struck an electrical light and caused it to break. The child was injured by the falling glass. The window pole normally would be considered to be a harmless instrument. In this instance, it led inadvertently to a situation in the classroom where a child was injured. Upon hearing this case, the court ruled that the school board must pay the costs for the injury to the student.

Not only have the courts held that the school board must maintain a safe and healthful school facility for children during the school day, but, also, it has been the opinion of the courts that the functions of a school district are not limited to just education of school children. The responsibility of the school board includes maintaining the school building for public meetings.

The importance of maintaining a healthful and safe school environment at times other than during the school day was emphasized in litigation in the state of California.[14] A woman slipped and broke her hip while going through the school foyer on her way to attend an educational lecture. She later brought suit against the school district. The floor of the foyer had been cleaned and waxed before the evening program. The suit charged that the woman was injured because the soap and wax mixture on the particular type of floor material presented an unsafe condition. The opinion of the court was that the soap and wax mixture should not have been used at all if its use created an unsafe environmental condition. It was felt that the floor was being maintained in a dangerous and defective condition. As a result, the court ruled that the school district was

---

14. Lorenz v. Santa Monica City High School Dist., et al., 124 P. 2d 846 (Calif., 1942).

negligent in not exercising ordinary care in the matter of providing a safe school environment.

A similar situation arose in New Jersey,[15] where a woman slipped on a highly waxed floor and was injured while attending a baton twirling exhibition at the school. The court ruled that in this situation such an activity, being sponsored by the school, must be considered a governmental function and, as such, the school board could not be found liable. However, of importance to the school health program was the fact that an improperly waxed and oiled school hallway caused an individual to slip and be injured. Such an environmental condition led to litigation. If the common law doctrine of governmental immunity had not been used in this case, a ruling of negligence very likely could have been rendered against the school district. This is very important today because the doctrine of governmental immunity is becoming less adhered to in several states.

Another situation in which litigation resulted from an accident to an individual while attending a nonschool-sponsored function occurred in Georgia.[16] In this case, a defective step was the cause for litigation. An individual had attended a dance recital at the school auditorium. The dance instructor had paid rental to the school for use of the auditorium. A woman was injured when she fell on a defective step. The court ruled that operation of the school auditorium was a governmental function even though the school district was receiving some income from the rental of the facility. As a governmental function, the concept of governmental

15. Thompson, *et ux. v.* Board of Education, City of Millville, 12 N.J. Super. 92, 79 A. 2d 100 (1951).

16. Smith *v.* Board of Education of City of Marietta, 167 S.E. 2d 615 (Ga., 1969).

immunity held and the school district was not held to be liable.

From the decisions rendered in these cases, two principles of law have been established. The schools are responsible not only for the normal educational activities of the school day, but, also, for providing a safe and healthy school environment which must be maintained for activities of a general public nature. A United States District Court in Pennsylvania[17] upheld this viewpoint in 1965. The second legal principle is that the school district, in providing a safe school environment, must not in turn produce a potentially more dangerous condition. When public schools are available for use by the general public, the school administration must have complete knowledge of the environmental conditions of the school building and grounds. Lack of knowledge concerning conditions of the school grounds, facilities, and building maintenance is considered to be negligent behavior on the part of school authorities. School authorities have a responsibility to know about potentially dangerous environmental conditions, and they must also see that correction of these conditions is made.

The schools not only have the responsibility for children while they are at school, but also a degree of responsibility rests with the schools for the children's welfare as they go to school and come home from school.

The importance of being responsible for students from the time they leave home until they return home means that the school bus transportation and the school safety patrol programs must be carefully planned and organized. It is the duty of the school district to provide extraordinary care for students going to and from school.

17. Rupe v. State Public School Building Authority, 245 F. Supp. 726 (Pa., 1965).

School Bus Transportation

The first provision for the transporting of school children occurred in Massachusetts in 1869. Since that time an ever increasing number of children have been riding school-provided transportation. As school districts become larger through school reorganization and consolidation, it will be necessary to transport more children to school every year by means of school buses. Legal control and direction for operation of the school bus transportation program can usually be found in the particular state statutes. It should be understood that school districts have no duty to supply transportation to their pupils unless such is required to be done by state statute. Authorization for providing school bus transportation is universally accepted in this country.

With the increasing number of students being carried to school on buses, a number of legal questions have arisen. Most commonly raised have been questions involving transporting pupils for the purpose of obtaining racial and ethnic balance in schools and litigations revolving around liability for injuries resulting to children while riding school buses. It is the latter question that shall be dealt with in this section.

The provision of transportation for the purpose of getting students to and from school has been ruled to be constitutional by the courts. In the past, many litigations resulted from people challenging the constitutionality of using tax money for the purpose of transporting children to school. In some states, mandatory statutes exist, requiring that the schools provide transportation for pupils. In other states, the statutes are of a permissive nature. In jurisdictions where statutes, rules, and regulations providing for the operation of a school bus transportation program have been challenged, the courts have ruled that the schools do have the authority to provide transportation for the students. The provision of transportation by the school district through the operation of a school bus program has been ruled to be a governmental function in numerous court opinions.[18]

For example, in 1964, a court in Iowa stated:

There can be no doubt the school district is an arm or agency of the state and that the maintenance of public schools, including providing transportation to the pupils entitled to it as required by statute, is a governmental function.[19]

It is important that the school administrator knows and follows the statutes regarding the school bus transportation program in the state in which he is located. A particular statute applicable in one state may not be legal in another state. Certainly it has little relevance to the school administrator in another state. If state statute should not provide for the school board to transport pupils, the courts are not agreed as to whether the school board can use public money for transportation of students to school. If the statute should be of a permissive nature, the decision is up to the school board as to whether transportation of pupils shall be provided.

Another question often raised in court litigation concerns who should be eligible for transportation to school and where is the bus required to pick up the students? Must

18. Bruggeman v. Independent School Dist. No. 4, Union Twp., Mitchell County, 289 N.W. 5 (Iowa, 1939). City of Bloomfield v. Davis County Community School District, 119 N.W. 2d 909 (Iowa, 1964). McKnight, et al. v. Cassady, et al., 174 A. 865 (N.J., 1934). Rittmiller v. School Dist. No. 84 (Wabasso County), et al., 104 F. Supp. 187 (Minn., 1952). Roberts v. Baker, et al., 196 S.E. 104 (Ga., 1938). Wallace v. Laurel County Board of Education, et al., 287 Ky. 454, 153 S.W. 2d 915 (1941).
19. City of Bloomfield v. Davis County Community School District, 119 N.W. 2d 912 (Iowa, 1964).

the school bus go to each child's house? How far are the children required to walk to meet the school bus? These are some of the questions that the individual school district must answer in light of the laws of its state and the rules and regulations of each particular state department of instruction. To serve as a guide to school administrators, various principles of law have been established by previous court decisions which can be of help in answering many of these questions when they are not established by state statute or regulation.

School districts may not necessarily be required to pick up each child at his own house. The courts have ruled that children may be required to walk a reasonable distance to meet the school bus. What distance can be considered reasonable walking distance varies from one area of the United States to another. Two miles was considered reasonable walking distance for children to go to meet a school bus in Kentucky.[20]

The courts have established in Indiana[21] that school buses do not have to go to the home of each pupil. Students may be required to travel a reasonable distance to meet a school bus. In 1958, a Wisconsin court[22] ruled that school buses do not have to go to the students' houses to pick up the children. The court suggested that students could be required to walk along a private road to meet the school bus at a common pick-up point. Students were required to walk as far as seven-tenths of a mile to meet the school bus.

This same concept was upheld in another case in Ken-

---

20. Board of Education of Clay County, et al. v. Bowling, et al., 312 Ky. 749, 229 S.W. 2d 769 (1950).
21. Lyle v. State ex rel Smith, 172 Ind. 502, 88 N.E. 850 (1909).
22. State ex rel. Miller, et al. v. Joint School Dist. No. 1, 5 Wis. 2d 16, 92 N.W. 2d 233 (1958).

tucky.[23] In this situation, three children, ages 8, 12, and 13, had to walk approximately one-half mile along a lightly traveled road to where the school bus picked them up. The father claimed that not only was the road dangerous to walk on, but it was "something of a 'lovers' lane' . . . children must walk past beer cans, whiskey bottles, mattresses, and other evidence of the road's use." The father further claimed that wild animals in the surrounding area were present which posed a danger to the children. Yet in court, no evidence could be presented that such animals were present in the particular area. The Court of Appeals of Kentucky ruled that requiring the children to walk the distance over the road in dispute was a reasonable regulation. The school board was not acting arbitrarily or unreasonably in refusing to send the school bus to the residence.

In establishing school bus routes, the courts usually will not interfere with the plans established by a school district if discretion is followed in setting up the routes. An Indiana case in 1923[24] supported this principle. School bus routes were to be determined by the school districts. It was ruled by the Indiana Supreme Court that the courts were not to direct by mandate the routes that the school vehicles were to take. This principle, that the courts will not interfere in the authority of the school district to establish a school bus route as long as it can be shown that proper discretion was being followed in the establishment of the routes, has been supported by courts in various other states.[25]

23. Hoefer v. Hardin County Board of Education, 441 S.W. 2d 418 (Ky., 1969).
24. State ex rel. Stewart, et al. v. Miller, 193 Ind. 492, 141 N.E. 60 (1923).
25. Pass, et al. v. Pickens, et al., 515 S.E. 2d 405 (Ga., 1949). State ex rel. Miller, et al. v. Joint School Dist. No. 1, supra. Woodlawn School Dist. No. 6 v. Brown, et al., 223 S.W. 2d 818 (Ark., 1949).

State statutes often provide that school children may be transported on a school bus if they live a given distance from the school. It is important that statutory requirement be followed regarding the distance from school the students must live before they are eligible to ride to school on school transportation. The required distance varies considerably from state to state. The standard normally accepted by the courts in determining distance to school is that of measuring the nearest traveled road that must be used in going to and from school.

A Mississippi statute stated that all children who live more than a mile from school should be provided with school bus transportation. In a very interesting court litigation,[26] the school board claimed that a particular family's children were not eligible for school bus transportation. The school claimed that the locations to be considered in determining the distance were to be measured from the end of the family driveway in front of their house to the point at school where the children were discharged from the bus. The parents of the children maintained that the distance must be measured from the front door of their house to the point at school where the children were discharged from the bus. A surveyor was asked to testify in this case. It was pointed out in court that the distance from the driveway to the school bus discharge point was 5,219.6 feet. The distance from the door of the house to the school was 5,364.6 feet. The court ruled that since the students lived in the house, and since it was found to be more than one mile from the house to the school bus discharge point, the school district must provide transportation to and from school for these children.

26. Madison County Board of Education *v.* Grantham, *et ux.*, 168 So. 2d 515 (Miss., 1964).

In a similar case in Wisconsin,[27] the court ruled that a family lived more than the required two mile limit specified in statute for being eligible to receive the benefits of school bus transportation. When the distance was originally measured, it was found that the distance between the student's house and the school building was eleven feet short of two miles. Therefore, the school district refused to permit the children to ride the school bus. Upon reconsideration, it was found that the distance was slightly over two miles, measured by the usually traveled route between the school and the home. Certain shortcuts taken in the original measurement were not considered to be part of the usually traveled route. The court ordered the school district to finance the transportation that the parents had been forced to pay between the two times that the measurements were conducted.

A number of litigations today involving affairs of school bus transportation are those concerning liability for injuries which result from accidents while the students are riding the school bus. As more pupils ride the buses, it becomes obvious that there is going to be an increase in the number of pupil injuries due to accidents involving school buses.

The defense of governmental immunity from tort liability has been applied to these matters the same as in any other aspect of the school program. Unless the state statute or common law has repealed the immunity for school bus situations, the doctrine of governmental immunity is in effect. With some states no longer adhering to the principle of governmental immunity, the consideration of liability of school bus transportation becomes ever more important.

School districts are responsible for the health, safety, and

---

27. Gandt v. Joint School Dist. No. 3 of the Towns of Oconto Falls, Morgan and Gillett, 4 Wis. 2d 419, 90 N.W. 2d 549 (1958).

well-being of the pupils while they are on the school bus. This principle was supported in a case in New York.[28] In this situation, a school district was sued for negligence in failing to properly equip the school bus with a heater. A fourteen year old girl's feet were frozen while riding the school bus. The court ruled in favor of the student, finding the school board negligent in failing to provide a properly equipped school bus.

Many cases of litigation have been brought against the school bus driver. The school bus driver is not immune from personal liability, even though he is employed by the school district. The school bus driver has a personal responsibility for all those who ride the bus. The importance of care and proper control of the school bus by the driver was emphasized in the following statement by a court in Louisiana:[29]

> While the highest degree of care, prudence and foresight is required of the operator of a school bus in receiving, carrying and discharging passengers and such an operator is liable to them for injuries occasioned by even the slightest negligence on his part, he does not insure the safety of his passengers, and there can be no liability in the absence of any negligence.

Because of the many dangers involved in transporting children to and from school, the school bus driver must be extremely careful. It is important that the individual driving the school bus always exercise extraordinary care whenever transporting school children. In making reference to the school bus driver, a court in New Jersey stated:[30]

---

28. Armlin v. Spickerman, et al., 250 App. Div. 810, 294 N.Y.S. 159 (1937).
29. Norris, et ux. v. American Casualty Company, et al., 176 So. 2d 678 (La., 1965).
30. Jackson v. Hankinson, 238 A. 2d 685 (N.J., 1968).

Where . . . they have provided transportation to and from school in a school bus . . . their obligation continues during the course of the transportation. If they negligently fail to discharge their duty . . . they should be held accountable in the same manner as other tortfeasors.

In a Georgia case,[31] a school bus driver was found liable for injuries to a pupil's eye. While riding the school bus, a tree limb entered an open window and struck a child's eye. Suit resulted and the court held that "school bus operators . . . are required to exercise extra-ordinary care for the safety of school children riding on their buses."

The question as to the place of the school bus driver in maintaining discipline on the school bus has not been answered clearly by court precedent. Does the school bus driver stand *in loco parentis* with respect to the children on the school bus?

It would seem to indicate from a 1957 case in New York[32] that a school bus driver has the legal right to discipline children who disobey on the school bus. In this case, a student refused to obey an order given by the school bus driver. As the result of the disobedience, a minor scuffle followed. In the opinion of the judge, the student was guilty of disorderly conduct by refusing to obey the instructions of the school bus driver. The court ruled that the driver had the right to correct the student's misbehavior.

Court cases involving school bus driver negligence in situations where the child becomes injured getting off the school bus are not infrequent. The most prevalent cases where pupils are injured with respect to school bus transportation have been associated with the loading and unloading of buses at the school and with accidents which

31. Eason *v.* Crews, 77 S.E. 2d 245 (Ga., 1953).
32. Neal: In re., 164 N.Y.S. 2d 549 (1957).

happen after children get off the bus and proceed from the bus to their homes. Leibee suggested several principles to be followed with respect to the matter of children getting off the bus. These principles are based upon decisions rendered by various courts of law:

1. The age of the pupil and his ability or lack of ability to look after himself is a dominant factor in determining the amount of care necessary.
2. The area of legal responsibility for the immature pupil extends beyond the mere unloading of the child in a safe place. It includes the known pathway the pupil must immediately pursue.
3. There is an imperative duty to warn proportionate to the child and to the conditions to warn.
4. It is the duty of drivers (bus) to see that pupils who must cross the road are in a place of safety before the drivers set the vehicle again in motion.
5. Contributory negligence is not acceptable as a defense in a case involving a child under seven (7) years of age.[33]

Not only must the school bus driver release a child in a safe location, but a Georgia Court of Appeals stated:[34]

It is the duty of a school-bus driver to deposit a passenger in a place of safety and, in the case of an infant, whether or not a place of deposit is a place of safety cannot be determined solely by whether or not one would be safe if he remained on that spot.

A nine year old child was involved in this Georgia case. It was the opinion of the court that the school bus driver was negligent in not rendering assistance to the boy. The boy was struck by a car as he attempted to leave the school

33. Howard C. Leibee, *Tort Liability for Injuries to Pupils* (Ann Arbor, Mich.: Campus Publishers, 1965), p. 67.
34. Davidson *v.* Horne, *et al.,* 71 S.E. 2d 468 (Ga., 1952).

bus and go to his home. The court ruling was based on the fact that the school bus driver was negligent in not following statutory regulations which required that he bring the bus to a stop at the far right side of the road.

In another Georgia case,[35] a child was killed by a passing vehicle after being deposited from the school bus. The court felt that the school bus driver had a duty to deposit the student at a reasonably safe location. However, it was the ruling of the court that the driver was under no obligation to warn students of the usual dangers of traffic each time that they got off the school bus.

In 1963, the Maryland Court of Appeals[36] rendered a decision that a school bus driver was properly supervising a discharged passenger's crossing the street if the student were with a school safety patrol. The use of school safety patrols for the purpose of helping students cross the street after getting off the bus was considered to be a reasonable action. In this particular case, an eight year old boy had gotten off the bus in the company of a school patrol. The patrol took the child to the edge of the bus and waited until the traffic was clear. The patrol then released the boy. The boy was hit by a car not seen until it was too late. The parents sued the bus driver, claiming lack of sufficient supervision. The court stated with respect to the school bus driver's responsibility to supervise the boy's crossing the street:

We think it was fulfilled by permitting the child to leave the bus in the company of a responsible student, a member of the safety patrol whose specific function was to shepherd younger children across the street. The use of such patrolmen is generally regarded as a reasonable and adequate provision for the safety of school bus riders.

35. Greeson v. Davis, et al., 9 S.E. 2d 690 (Ga., 1940).
36. Ragonese v. Hilferty, 191 A. 2d 422 (Md., 1963).

School Safety Patrol

The school safety patrol has developed into an integral part of the school program. With the rise in number of automobiles, the importance of this school service has expanded greatly. The purposes of the school safety patrol must be extremely clear and serve as a guide in the organization and planning of this program. The major purposes of a school safety patrol should be educational in nature. The most commonly expressed objectives of the school safety patrol program are: 1) to control pedestrian traffic of school children, 2) to teach safety understandings, 3) to develop certain safety habits, and 4) to teach good citizenship.

Because of the possibility of injury to students involved in the school safety patrol program, it is very important that proper planning, organization, administration, and close supervision of the program be carried out. Such practices as permitting the patrol members to direct vehicular traffic and allowing them to enter the streets to perform their duties must be forbidden.

At least thirteen of the fifty states have statutes which provide in some way for a school safety patrol program. No state has a statute which would prohibit a school safety patrol.

TABLE 7 *States Having Statutory Provision Authorizing a School Safety Patrol*

Alaska	New Jersey
Idaho	New York
Massachusetts	Pennsylvania
Michigan	Utah
Minnesota	Vermont
Mississippi	Wisconsin
Montana	

Legal precedent would appear to suggest that unless required by statute, a school district does not have to provide a school safety patrol. This was the ruling in a court case in California[37] where it was found not to be mandatory that the school district furnish a school safety patrol. In this situation, a five-year-old boy was struck by a car near the school about noon. His father claimed that the school district was negligent through their failure to provide protection for the children at a busy intersection. Safety patrol members had been removed by the school authorities as a result of protests by some parents. The court ruled that the school district could not be held liable for failing to furnish a safety patrol in the absence of some statute making such action mandatory.

The importance of careful selection and training of school safety patrol members was emphasized in an Indiana Attorney General's opinion handed down in 1929. The attorney general stated that school officials were not liable for the actions of students involved as school safety patrols. It was the opinion of the attorney general that the schools could not require pupils to serve on the school patrol. Service on the school safety patrol must be voluntary. Not only must service on the safety patrol be voluntary, but reasonable care must be used in selecting patrol members. The consent of a student's parents or guardian should be given before a child is permitted to serve on the patrol. All of these concepts are supported to some degree by the various state statutes authorizing organization of a safety patrol.

In authorizing the schools of Alaska to establish a safety patrol, that state legislature made consultation with local

---

37. Wright *v.* Arcade School District, 40 Calif. Rptr. 812 (1964).

law enforcement authorities a requirement. In Idaho, a school safety patrol member may report any vehicular violation observed while on duty.

Careful instructions, rules, and regulations must be known, understood, and followed by all patrol members. If proper precautions are taken by the school authorities, it is doubtful that a school administrator or other school personnel would be found negligent regarding matters involving the safety patrol. It would seem that the following procedures are necessary to protect the sponsoring teacher or school administrator from danger of liability with respect to the school safety patrol program: 1) service on the school safety patrol must be voluntary and not mandatory, 2) extreme care must be taken in the selection of patrol members, 3) parental permission must be given before a child is permitted to serve on the patrol, and 4) specific instruction in duties must be carefully given, fully understood, and followed.

An interesting observation is that to date no court case is known to have been brought against a school administrator or other school personnel in which he or she was found liable in matters involving the school safety patrol.

The National Commission on Safety Education has suggested the following standards for formulating a school safety patrol:

1. The school superintendent should assume the leadership in determining over-all school safety patrol policies.
2. Careful instruction and continuous supervision of the patrols by qualified and responsible school personnel are essential.
3. All patrol members should be properly instructed in their duties and given "on-the-job" training before being assigned.
4. Members of the safety patrols should be selected from the upper grades, preferably not below the fifth, on the basis of their leadership and reliability.

5. Patrol services should be voluntary and open to all who qualify; written approval of the parents should be secured.[38]

Several agencies are available that will help to develop guidelines for school administrators to follow in establishing a school safety patrol. Examples of such agencies are the National Safety Council, the American Automobile Association, the National Education Association, the National Congress of Parents and Teachers, and the United States Office of Education.

Summary

The school district has an obligation to provide a safe and healthful school environment. Since school children legally are required to attend school, it must be assumed that they will have provided for them an environment which is safe and conducive to good health. Not only is the school district responsible for the health and well-being of school children while they are on the school grounds, but, also, there is a responsibility for these children as they come to the school and return home.

In providing a safe school environment, the school district must not, in turn, produce a potentially more dangerous environmental condition. It is the responsibility of all school personnel (administrators, teachers, custodial staff, and others) to be aware of any potentially dangerous conditions on the school grounds. Lack of knowledge by school personnel regarding conditions on the school grounds, facilities, and buildings, is considered to be negligent behavior. Not only must school personnel be aware of any potentially dangerous conditions on the school grounds, but if condi-

---

38. National Commission on Safety Education, *Who Is Liable for Pupil Injury?* (Washington, D.C.: National Education Assoc., 1963), p. 61.

tions warrant correction, steps must be taken to implement such changes immediately. Failure to make some degree of effort to correct dangerous environmental conditions has been shown by the courts to be an act of negligence.

School districts are responsible for maintaining a safe and healthful environment of the school facilities for activities of a general public nature in addition to regular school day activities.

School districts have been involved in an extensive number of litigations regarding the school bus transportation program. The operation of a school bus transportation program has been found to be constitutional and has been ruled to be a governmental function rather than a proprietary function. There is a responsibility on the part of the school board to provide a healthful environment for children as they ride the school bus. The school bus does not have to go directly to the home of the students. Children may be required to walk a reasonable distance for the purpose of meeting the bus. In determining distance from a child's house to the school for the purpose of establishing his eligibility to ride the school bus, the distance shall be measured over the nearest traveled road that is taken by the school bus.

The school bus driver is not immune from personal liability for his actions while operating the bus. This individual has a moral and legal responsibility to the children for their safety and welfare while on the bus.

The school safety patrol has been established in many schools for the purpose of assisting the children in going to and from school. Unless provided for by statute, the school does not have to furnish a school safety patrol. School safety patrol programs must be well planned, organized, and closely supervised. Service on the school safety patrol must be voluntary. Permission to serve on the patrol should be given by the student's parents or guardian. It is extremely important that potential school safety patrol members be instructed concerning their duties and responsibilities.

The provision of a healthful school environment must be for the purpose of aiding students to benefit more fully from their educational experiences. Such provision has been upheld by statutes and attorney generals' opinions, as well as in court decisions throughout the United States.

9

The School Lunch Program

For many years, the provision of a lunch program by the schools has been considered to be an important part of the educational program. It has been felt that this program contributes to the total education of school children. The school lunch program can be an area of potential litigation for the school district. The two leading questions that have resulted in court litigations are in matters concerning tort liability in the operation of the program and in questions concerning whether operation of the school lunch program is a governmental function or a commercial enterprise.

The courts have ruled that operation of a school lunch program is a governmental function. As such, the schools have every legal right to operate such a program. This principle has been established on the premise that the school lunch program is conducted for the purpose of contributing to the health and welfare of the students. Operation of such a program must not be conducted for profit.

Suit has been brought several times against school districts by proprietors of restaurants, claiming that the feeding of children at school deprived the restaurant owners of a vital source of personal revenue. These cases usually have

138

claimed that operation of a school lunch program was in competition with and injurious to their businesses. The school districts were challenged on the grounds that as a governmental agency whose purpose it was to educate young people, there was no reason why a noon lunch program should be operated. The schools were to educate, not feed the students, was the rationale usually put forth by those raising opposition to such programs.

Suit was brought against a school district in Denver[1] because the schools were operating lunch rooms. Students, teachers, school employees, and visitors were eating at the school instead of frequenting the neighboring restaurant. This lawsuit charged that such activity deprived the restaurant owner of his major source of income. Because of the operation of the school lunch program, school children no longer ate at his restaurant. The restaurant owner claimed that this was an invasion of private property by a governmental agency. In ruling on this case the United States Circuit Court of Appeals made the following statement:

> The school board does not conduct these cafeterias for profit, and in commercial competition with private restaurants and eating houses. The students are kept in during the lunch hour for reasons which intimately concern their welfare as students. . . . The cafeterias are necessary conveniences. Opportunity is thus afforded to the students to enjoy well selected, well prepared, and nourishing food, adapted to their needs. The amount charged is only for the purpose of maintaining these facilities and not for commercial profit. In many cases it is impracticable for the students to reach home and return within time for a proper enjoyment of food. The practice has for its object the physical welfare of the students, which is an important factor in their educational development.

1. Goodman v. School District No. 1, City and County of Denver, et al., 32 F. 2d 586 (Colo., 1929).

The court recognized that it was conceivable that the practice of operating a lunch program in the schools could be abused. However, operation of such a program was felt to be constitutional and did not deprive the restaurant owner of his primary source of income. Similar opinions have been rendered in various other states.

The schools often require that school children must eat their lunch at school. The students are not permitted to leave the building during the lunch recess. In a case in New York,[2] the court ruled that school boards have the authority to adopt rules and regulations which they feel are necessary for the orderly operation of a school program. It was held in this case that the courts should not interfere with such rules and regulations unless it could be shown that the ruling was made in an arbitrary manner. Requiring students to eat their lunches in the school cafeteria was held to be a legal ruling and not an arbitrary act on the part of the school board.

In another situation which resulted in litigation,[3] the principal passed a regulation prohibiting school children from entering a restaurant adjacent to the school grounds during the school hours of 8:15 a.m. and 3:00 p.m. The school furnished lunches in the school lunchroom for all students. Upon request from their parents, children were permitted to go home for lunch.

Suit was brought against the school, claiming that the ruling which prohibited students from entering the adjacent restaurant was not legal. The circuit court ruled that the school regulation was void. However, in appeal to the state court of appeals, the decision was reversed and the school

2. Fitzpatrick *v.* Board of Education of Central School District No. 2 of the Town of St. Johnsville, 284 N.Y.S. 2d 590 (1967).
3. Casey County Board of Education, *et al. v.* Luster, *et al.*, 282 S.W. 2d 333 (Ky., 1955).

ruling was held to be legal. Basis for the higher court's decision rested on the principle that public schools may make and enforce regulations which are considered to be reasonable for the actual management and control of the school program.

The school board cannot lease school land to an individual for the purpose of building a cafeteria to feed school children. A school district in Louisiana[4] was planning to lease to an individual a portion of land owned by the school district. This individual was going to build an eating establishment for the purpose of feeding school children and school personnel. The court ruled against this action. The decision of the court was based mainly on the fact that the school board would have had no direct control over the cafeteria. Also, the owner of the cafeteria gave no indication that he would sell food and lunches to school pupils and teachers only.

Litigation concerning tort liability in the operation of the school lunch program has not been common. Part of the reason for this may be because the operation of the school lunch program has been declared by the courts to be a governmental function and, therefore, probably a school district would be found to be immune from tort liability based upon the common law doctrine of governmental immunity.

An example of this was a case in Ohio[5] which involved a student who was eating a hamburger at school. One bite of the sandwich contained a large piece of metal. The child's throat was injured as the result of swallowing the piece of metal. The school board was sued by the parents who contended that the school was negligent in failing

4. Presley v. Vernon Parish School Board, 19 La. Ap. 217, 139 So. 692 (1932).
5. Elias v. Norton, et al., 53 Ohio App. 38, 4 N.E. 2d 146 (1936).

to maintain the cafeteria in a clean and sanitary condition. The court found that the board of education was not liable for damages to this student because operation of the lunchroom was a governmental function authorized by state statute. With the gradual changing of the concept of governmental immunity as it relates to school districts, it is important that all school administrators be alert to those possibilities for litigation in the operation of the school lunch programs.

Twenty-three states have some statutory provisions authorizing the local school district to establish a school lunch service program. In these states, the statute usually is of a permissive nature. The local school board is given permission to establish such a program. Usually the statute authorizes employment of personnel, the purchase of equipment and supplies, and the using of specified money to operate the program. In most statutes, the individual state legislature has authorized the state department of education to accept federal money to be used in the school lunch program.

TABLE 8 *States Authorizing School Lunch Programs by State Statute*

Arizona	Michigan
California	Missouri
Colorado	Montana
Connecticut	North Dakota
Georgia	Ohio
Illinois	Oregon
Indiana	Pennsylvania
Iowa	Rhode Island
Kansas	Utah
Louisiana	Vermont
Maine	Wyoming
Massachusetts	

In a somewhat unusual provision, the state of Utah has a statute which says that a tax on retail sale of wine and distilled liquors in the state shall be collected for the purpose of funding the school lunch program.

One state, Georgia, goes beyond simply authorizing the establishment of the school lunch program, and suggests in statutory provision that the local school district may include instruction in nutrition, hygiene, etiquette, and the "social graces" relating to the partaking of meals. It further recommends that school cafeterias, school lunch personnel, and other school staff be used in this program.

The California state legislature has passed the Duffy-Moscone Family Nutrition Education and Services Act of 1970. This Act established an ongoing program to assure adequate nutritional requirements of pupils in receipt of public assistance. Breakfast and lunch is to be provided at school for children from poor families. The intent of this program is to be of more than a nutritive value for the children. It is intended to also include the parents of the children. The parents are to be involved in the planning, preparation, and serving of the meals at the school. A nominal cash payment may be required of not less than five cents per meal nor more than twenty cents per meal. Milk is to be included at each meal.

In recent years, other programs have been developed in many states for the purpose of providing meals for children of indigent circumstances. Not only is a noon meal provided in many localities, but many school districts now provide a breakfast for certain needy children. This represents a change in attitude from legal opinion of some years ago. In a case in Louisiana,[6] the operation of a school lunch

6. Ralph v. Orleans Parish School Board, 158 La. 659, 104 So. 490 (1925).

program was found to be legal. However, the Supreme Court of Louisiana emphasized that such meals for students and teachers should be available during the noon lunch hours only. Today this concept is of doubtful consequence.

Summary

The school lunch program must be considered a contributing factor in the educational development of the school child. This program is considered to be a part of the total school program and, as such, has been declared a governmental function. The courts have upheld the right of schools to require that students remain at school during the lunch period. The operation of a school lunch program has been shown not to be in conflict with private restaurants.

Summary of Court Cases

Alabama

Mitchell *v.* McCall, *et al.*, 143 So. 2d 629 (1962).

Arizona

Globe School Dist. No. 1, of Globe, Gila County *v.* Board of Health of City of Globe, 20 Ariz. 208, 179 P. 55 (1919).

Arkansas

Allen, *et al. v.* Ingalls, *et al.*, 182 Ark. 991, 33 S.W. 2d 1099 (1930).

Auten *v.* Board of Directors of Special School District of Little Rock, 83 Ark. 431, 104 S.W. 130 (1907).

Cude *v.* State, 377 S.W. 2d 816 (1964).

Mannis *v.* State *ex rel.* DeWitt School District #1, 398 S.W. 2d 206 (1966).

Woodlawn School Dist. No. 6 *v.* Brown, *et al.*, 223 S.W. 2d 818 (1949).

Wright *v.* DeWitt School Dist. No. 1 of Arkansas County, 385 S.W. 2d 644 (1965).

California

Andre, *et al.* *v.* Allyn, *et al.*, 190 P. 2d 949 (1948).

Eastham *v.* Santa Clara Elementary School District, 76 Cal. Rptr. 198 (1969).

Lehmuth *v.* Long Beach Unified School District, *et al.*, 343 P. 2d 422 (1959).

Lilienthal *v.* The San Leandro Unified School District of Alameda County, 293 P. 2d 889 (1956).

Lorenz *v.* Santa Monica City High School Dist., *et al.*, 124 P. 2d 846 (1942).

Ogando *v.* Carquinez Grammar School District of Contra Costa County, *et al.*, 24 Calif. App. 2d 567, 75 P. 2d 641 (1938).

Pirkle *v.* Oakdale Union Grammar School District, City of Oakland, County of Stanislaus, 40 Cal. 2d 207, 253 P. 2d 1 (1953).

State Board of Health *v.* Board of Trustees of Watsonville School Dist. of Santa Cruz County, *et al.*, 13 Calif. App. 514, 110 P. 137 (1910).

Welch *v.* Dunsmuir Joint Union High School District, 326 P. 2d 633 (1958).

Wright *v.* Arcade School District, 40 Cal. Rptr. 812 (1964).

Colorado

Flemming *v.* Colorado State Board of Education, 400 P. 2d 932 (1965).

Goodman *v.* School District No. 1, City and County of Denver, *et al.*, 32 F. 2d 586 (1929).

Hallett, *et al.* *v.* Post Printing and Publishing Co., 68 Colo. 573, 192 P. 658 (1920).

Georgia

Davidson *v.* Horne, *et al.*, 866 Ga. App. 220, 71 S.E. 2d 464 (1952).

Eason *v.* Crews, 88 Ga. App. 602, 77 S.E. 2d 245 (1953).

Greeson *v.* Davis, *et al.,* 9 S.E. 2d 690 (1940).

Pass, *et al. v.* Pickens, *et al.,* 515 S.E. 2d 405 (1949).

Roberts *v.* Baker, *et al.,* 196 S.E. 104 (1938).

Smith *v.* Board of Education of City of Marietta, 167 S.E. 2d 615 (1969).

Hawaii

Medeiros *v.* Kiyosaki, 478 P. 2d 314 (1970).

Illinois

Board of Education of the City of Rockford *v.* Page, *et al.,* 33 Ill. 2d 372, 211 N.E. 2d 361 (1965).

Molitor *v.* Kaneland Community Unit District No. 302, 163 N.E. 2d 89 (1959).

Indiana

Blue *v.* Beach, 155 Ind. 121, 56 N.E. 89 (1900).

Fertich *v.* Michener, 111 Ind. 472, 11 N.E. 605 (1887).

Gamble, *et al. v.* Lewis, 227 Ind. 455, 85 N.E. 2d 629 (1949).

Lyle *v.* State *ex rel.* Smith, 172 Ind. 502, 88 N.E. 850 (1909).

State *ex rel.* Andrews *v.* Webber, 108 Ind. 31, 8 N.E. 708 (1886).

State *ex rel.* Horne *v.* Beil, *et al.,* 60 N.E. 672 (1901).

State *ex rel.* Stewart *v.* Miller, 193 Ind. 492, 141 N.E. 60 (1923).

Vonnegut *v.* Baum, 206 Ind. 172, 188 N.E. 677 (1934).

Iowa

Bruggeman *v.* Independent School Dist. No. 4, Union Twp., Mitchell County, 289 N.W. 5 (1939).

City of Bloomfield *v.* Davis County Community School District, 119 N.W. 2d 909 (1963).

Valentine *v.* Independent School Dist. of Casey, *et al.*, 174 N.W. 334 (1919).

Kentucky

Board of Education of Bowling Green *v.* Simmons, 53 S.W. 2d 940 (1932).

Board of Education of Clay County, *et al. v.* Bowling, *et al.*, 312 Ky. 749, 229 S.W. 2d 769 (1950).

Casey County Board of Education, *et al. v.* Luster, *et al.*, 282 S.W. 2d 333 (1955).

Hoefer *v.* Hardin County Board of Education, 441 S.W. 2d 418 (1969).

Lawson, *et al. v.* Commonwealth, 291 Ky. 437, 164 S.W. 2d 972 (1942).

Wallace *v.* Laurel County Board of Education, *et al.*, 287 Ky. 454, 153 S.W. 2d 915 (1941).

Louisiana

Norris, *et ux. v.* American Casualty Company, *et al.*, 176 So. 2d 677 (1965).

Presley *v.* Vernon Parish School Board, 19 La. Ap. 217, 139 So. 692 (1932).

Ralph *v.* Orleans Parish School Board, 158 La. 659, 104 So. 490 (1925).

Maryland

Cornwell *v.* State Board of Education, 314 F. Supp. 340, affirmed 428 F. 2d 471 (1969).

Ragonese *v.* Hilferty, 231 Md. 520, 191 A. 2d 422 (1963).

Massachusetts

Commonwealth *v.* Green, 268 Mass. 585, 168 N.E. 101 (1929).

Jacobson *v.* Commonwealth of Massachusetts, 197 U.S. 11, 255 S. Ct. 358, 49 L. Ed. 643 (1905).

Molinari *v.* The City of Boston, 130 N.E. 2d 925 (1955).

Mower *v.* The Inhabitants of Leicester, 9 Mass. 247 (1812).

Michigan

People *ex rel.* Hill *v.* Board of Education of City of Lansing, *et al.*, 224 Mich. 388, 195 N.W. 95 (1923).

Minnesota

Bang *v.* Independent School Dist. No. 27 of St. Louis County, 225 N.W. 449 (1929).

Rittmiller *v.* School Dist. No. 84 (Wabasso County), *et al.*, 104 F. Supp. 187 (1952).

State *ex rel.* Stoltenberg *v.* Brown, 112 Minn. 370, 128 N.W. 294 (1910).

Stone *v.* Probst, *et al.*, 165 Minn. 361, 206 N.W. 642 (1925).

Mississippi

Madison County Board of Education *v.* Grantham, *et ux.*, 168 So. 2d 515 (1964).

Nebraska

Odom *v.* Willms, 131 N.W. 2d 140 (1964).

New Hampshire

State *v.* Drew, 192 A. 629 (1937).

New Jersey

Board of Education of Mountain Lakes *v.* Maas, 56 N.J. Super. 245, 152 A. 2d 394 (1959).

Duda, *et al. v.* Gaines, *et al.*, 12 N.J. Super. 326, 79 A. 2d 695 (1951).

Jackson *v.* Hankinson, 51 N.J. 230, 238 A. 2d 685 (1968).

Kolbeck *v.* Kramer, 84 N.J. Super. 569, 202 A. 2d 889 (1964).

McKnight, *et al. v.* Cassady, *et al.*, 174 A. 865 (1934).

Thompson, *et ux. v.* Board of Education, City of Millville, 12 N.J. Super. 92, 79 A. 2d 100 (1951).

Valent *v.* New Jersey State Board of Education, 274 A. 2d 832 (1971).

New Mexico

Bourne *v.* Board of Education of City of Roswell, 46 N.M. 310, 128 P. 2d 733 (1942).

New York

Applebaum *v.* Board of Education of City of New York, 297 N.Y. 762, 77 N.E. 2d 785 (1948).

Armlin *v.* Spickerman, *et al.*, 250 App. Div. 810, 294 N.Y.S. 159 (1937).

Corlov *v.* Nyquest, 304 N.Y.S. 2d 486 (1969).

Corsover *v.* Board of Examiners of City of New York, 298 N.Y.S. 2d 757 (1968).

Elwell, In re., 284 N.Y.S. 2d 924 (1967).

Feuerstein *v.* Board of Education of the City of New York, 202 N.Y.S. 2d 524 (1960).

Fitzpatrick *v.* Board of Education of Central School District No. 2 of the Town of St. Johnsville, 284 N.Y.S. 2d 590 (1967).

Gardner v. State of New York, 10 N.Y.S. 274 (1939).

Hovey v. State, 261 App. Civ. 759, 27 N.Y.S. 2d 195 (1941).

Johnson v. Board of Education of the City of New York, 220 N.Y.S. 2d 362 (1961).

Kropf v. Board of Education of City of New York, 238 N.Y.S. 2d 757 (1963).

McCartney, et al. v. Austin, et al., 298 N.Y.S. 2d 26 (1969).

Miller v. Board of Education, Union Free School, Dist. No. 1, of Town of Albion, et al., 291 N.Y. 25, 50 N.E. 2d 529 (1943).

Neal, In re., 164 N.Y.S. 2d 549 (1957).

Peck v. Board of Education of City of Mount Vernon, et al., 317 N.Y.S. 2d 919 (1970).

Popow v. Central School Dist. No. 1, et al., 251 App. Div. 906, 297 N.Y.S. 205 (1937).

VanAllen v. McCleary, 211 N.Y.S. 2d 501 (1961).

Young v. City of New York, et al., 307 N.Y.S. 2d 576 (1970).

North Carolina

State v. Miday, 140 S.E. 2d 325 (1966).

State v. Pendergrass, 19 N.C. 348 (1837).

North Dakota

Martin v. Craig, et al., 42 N.D. 213, 173 N.W. 787 (1919).

Rhea v. Board of Education of Devils Lake Special School District, 41 N.D. 449, 171 N.W. 103 (1919).

Ohio

Elias v. Norton, et al., 53 Ohio App. 38, 4 N.E. 2d 146 (1936).

State ex rel. Mack v. Board of Education of Covington, 1 Ohio App. 2d 143, 204 N.E. 2d 86 (1963).

Oregon

Lovell *v.* School District No. 13, Coos County, 143 P. 2d 236 (1943).

School Board of School District No. U2-20 Jt., Multnomah County *v.* Fanning, 377 P. 2d 4 (1962).

Pennsylvania

Duffield *v.* School District of City of Williamsport, 162 Pa. 476, 29 A. 742 (1894).

Lee *v.* Marsh, 230 Pa. 351, 79 A. 564 (1911).

Lyndall *v.* High School Committee, 19 Pa. Super. Ct. 232 (1901).

Marsh, In re., 140 Pa. Super. 472, 14 A. 2d 368 (1940).

Rupe *v.* State Public School Building Authority, 245 Fed. Supp. 726 (1965).

Supler *v.* School District of North Franklin Township, Washington County, 182 A. 2d 535 (1962).

South Dakota

Streich *v.* Board of Education of Independent School Dist. of City of Aberdeen, *et al.*, 34 S.D. 169, 147 N.W. 779 (1914).

Tennessee

Reed *v.* Rhea County, 225 S.W. 2d 49 (1949).

Texas

Abney *v.* Fox, *et al.*, 250 S.W. 210 (1923).

Morris *v.* Smiley, *et al.*, 378 S.W. 2d 149 (1964).

Moseley, *et al. v.* City of Dallas, *et al.*, 17 S.W. 2d 36 (1929).

West Virginia

Jarrett *v.* Goodall, 113 W. Va. 478, 168 S.E. 763 (1933).

Wisconsin

Gandt *v.* Joint School Dist. No. 3 of the Towns of Oconto Falls, Morgan and Gillett, 4 Wis. 2d 419, 90 N.W. 2d 549 (1958).

State *ex rel.* Adams *v.* Burdge, *et al.*, 70 N.W. 347 (1897).

State *ex rel.* Miller, *et al. v.* Joint School Dist. No. 1, 5 Wis. 2d 16, 92 N.W. 2d 233 (1958).

Foreign

Russell *v.* The Men Dwelling in the County of Devon, 100 Eng. Rep. 359, 2 Term Rep. 671 (1788).

Bibliography

Legal Encyclopedias and Legal References

American Digest System. West Publishing Co., St. Paul, Minn., Century Edition, 1658 to 1896; Decennial Edition, 1897 to 1906; Second Decennial Edition, 1907 to 1916; Third Decennial Edition, 1916 to 1926; Fourth Decennial Edition, 1926 to 1936; Fifth Decennial Edition, 1936 to 1946; Sixth Decennial Edition, 1946 to 1956; Seventh Decennial Edition, 1956 to 1966.

American Jurisprudence. Rochester, N.Y.: The Lawyers Cooperative Publishing Co., 1943; with supplement, 1971.

Black, Henry Campbell. *Black's Law Dictionary.* St. Paul, Minn.: West Publishing Co., 1951, 1882 pp.

Corpus Juris. London: The American Law Book, Co., 1932.

Corpus Juris Secundum. Brooklyn, N.Y.: The American Law Book Co., 1952; with supplement, 1971.

National Reporter System. West Publishing Co., St. Paul, Minn., continuous since 1879.
Atlantic Reporter
Atlantic Reporter, Second Series
Federal Reporter
Federal Reporter, Second Series
New York Supplement
New York Supplement, Second Series
Northeastern Reporter
Northeastern Reporter, Second Series

Northwestern Reporter
Northwestern Reporter, Second Series
Pacific Reporter
Pacific Reporter, Second Series
Southeastern Reporter
Southeastern Reporter, Second Series
Southern Reporter
Southern Reporter, Second Series
Southwestern Reporter
Southwestern Reporter, Second Series
Supreme Court Reporter

Shepherd's Citations, The Frank Shepard Company, New York.
Atlantic Reporter Citations
Federal Reporter Citations
New York Supplement Citations
Northeastern Reporter Citations
Northwestern Reporter Citations
Pacific Reporter Citations
Southeastern Reporter Citations
Southern Reporter Citations
Southwestern Reporter Citations
United States Citations

West's General Digest, Fourth Series. Vols. 1-17. St. Paul, Minn.:
West Publishing Co., 1967-1971.

Books

Baker, Robert E. *The Implications of School Liability for Teach-
ers of Health (Physical) Education in New York City.* New
York, N.Y.: Unpublished Doctor's Thesis, Advanced School
of Education, Teacher College, Columbia University, 1956,
163 pp., typed.
Bucher, Charles A. *Administration of School and College Health
and Physical Education Programs.* St. Louis, Mo.: The
C. V. Mosby Co., 1967, 671 pp.
Bund, Emanuel, Editor. *The Education Court Digest.* New
York: Published by Emanuel Bund, 1957-1964.

Burt, Lorin A. *School Law and the Indiana Teacher.* Bloomington, Ind.: Beanblossom Publishers, 1967.

Byrd, Oliver E. *School Health Administration.* Philadelphia:
W. B. Saunders Co., 1964, 491 pp.

Constantine, Gus A. *Legal Liability for Injuries Sustained in
the Transportation of Public School Pupils.* Durham, N.C.:
Unpublished Doctor's Thesis, Duke University, 1958, 216
pp., typed.

Drury, Robert L. *Law and the School Superintendent.* Cincinnati, O: The W. H. Anderson Company, 1958, 339 pp.

Drury, Robert L. and Ray, Kenneth C. *Principles of School Law.*
New York: Appleton-Century-Crofts, 1965, 356 pp.

Edwards, Newton. *The Courts and the Public Schools.* Chicago:
University of Chicago Press, 1955, 622 pp.

Flowers, Ann and Bolmeier, Edward C. *Law and Pupil Control.*
Cincinnati, O.: The W. H. Anderson Company, 1964, 194 pp.

Fulbright, Evelyn R. and Bolmeier, Edward C. *Courts and the
Curriculum.* Cincinnati, O.: The W. H. Anderson Company,
1964, 197 pp.

Garber, Lee O. and Reutter, E. Edmund, Co-editors. *The Yearbook of School Law.* Danville, Ill.: The Interstate Printers
and Publishers, Inc., 1933-1971, annual.

Gauerke, Warren E. *School Law.* New York: The Center for
Applied Research in Education, Inc., 1965, 116 pp.

Grieve, Andrew W. *The Legal Aspects of Athletics.* Cranbury,
N.J.: A. S. Barnes and Company, Inc., 1969, 183 pp.

Hamilton, Otto Templar. *The Courts and the Curriculum.*
New York: Teachers College, Columbia University, 1927,
168 pp.

Leibee, Howard C. *Tort Liability for Injuries to Pupils.* Ann
Arbor, Mich.: Campus Publishers, 1965, 97 pp.

Mayshark, Cyrus and Shaw, Donald D. *Administration of School
Health Programs: Its Theory and Practice.* St. Louis, Mo.:
The C. V. Mosby Co., 1967, 483 pp.

National Education Association Research Division. *The Pupil's
Day in Court.* Washington, D.C.: National Education Association, 1958-1963, published annually.

————. *The Teacher's Day in Court.* Washington, D.C.: National Education Association, 1958-1963, published annually.

————. *Who Is Liable for Pupil Injuries?* Washington, D.C.: National Commission on Safety Education, National Education Association, 1963, 72 pp.

Nolte, M. Chester and Linn, John Phillip. *School Law For Teachers.* Danville, Ill.: The Interstate Printers and Publishers, Inc., 1963, 343 pp.

Notz, Rebecca Laurens Love. *Legal Bibliography and Legal Research.* Washington, D.C.: National Law Book Company, 1947, 234 pp.

Pollack, Ervin H. *Fundamentals of Legal Research.* Brooklyn, N.Y.: The Foundation Press, Inc., 1956, 295 pp.

Remmlein, Madaline Kinter. *School Law.* New York: McGraw-Hill Book Co., Inc., 1950, 376 pp.

Seitz, Reynolds C., Editor. *Law and The School Principal.* Cincinnati, O.: The W. H. Anderson Company, 1961, 266 pp.

Periodical References

Bolmeier, E. C. "Trends in Pupil Transportation Litigation," *The American School Board Journal* (February 1960). 140:38–40.

Fuller, Edgar. "Liability for Negligence of Educational Officers and Employees," *The American School Board Journal* (October and November 1941). 103:23–25; 29–30.

Garber, Lee O. "Several Principles of Law Affect Pupil Transportation," *The Nation's Schools* (August 1962). 62:41–2.

Garber, Lee O. and Evangelou, Van S. "Legal Problems Ride the School Bus," *The Nation's Schools* (April 1957). 59:85–9.

Hunter, Adelaide M.; Ortiz, Robert; and Martinez, Joe. "Compulsory and Voluntary School Immunization Programs in the United States," *Journal of School Health* (March 1963). 33:98–102.

Marconnit, George D. "State Legislatures and the School Curriculum," *Phi Delta Kappan* (January 1968). 49:269–72.

Miller, Dean F. "Legal Bases for School Health Practices in Indiana." *Journal of School Health* (October 1970). 40:446–50.

————. "Recent Litigations Involving the School Health Services." *Journal of School Health* (December 1970). 40:526–27.

Nolte, M. Chester. "Legal Implications in School Programs." *The American School Board Journal* (December 1964). 149:29.

"Schools and School Districts—Negligence—State Liability for Torts." *Indiana Law Journal* (February 1929). 4:343.

Seeley, Darwin. "School Accidents and Teacher Liability." *Journal of School Health* (May 1962). 32:190–91.

Shapiro, Frieda S. "Your Liability for Student Accidents." *Journal of the National Education Association* (March 1965). 54:46–7.

Trubitt, Hillard J. "Legal Responsibilities of School Teachers in Emergency Situations." *Journal of School Health* (January 1966). 36:22–8.

Index

159

DATE DUE

APR 22

30 505 JOSTEN'